AF223896

More Praise

As a psychologist, I live for days like this, although as you can well imagine, there's never been a day quite like this – after forty years! Wow. I am overjoyed for dear Cathy and so proud of her resilience.

— Céline Paris
Psychologist, Stroke Rehabilitation Team
Saint-Vincent Hospital, 1984

* * *

In November 2023, the Ottawa Citizen ran my column about why some stroke rehabilitation patients do well and others don't, where I outlined six points illustrating why geriatric rockers The Rolling Stones can continue to perform live and excite millions of people around the world.

Cathy's subsequent reply, comparing her own personal experiences with stroke, which also appeared in the Citizen one week later, was terrific. It made so much sense. Bruyère is now the primary provider of Stroke Rehabilitation in Ottawa, and I'm delighted she accepted my invitation to hold her book launch/ fundraising effort for the Bruyère Foundation.

— Dr. Hillel M. Finestone
Director of Stroke Rehabilitation Research, Bruyère Continuing Care, Élisabeth Bruyère Hospital and Professor, Physical Medicine and Rehabilitation, Department of Medicine, University of Ottawa

BECOMING COMFORTABLY NUMB

A MEMOIR ON BRAIN-MENDING

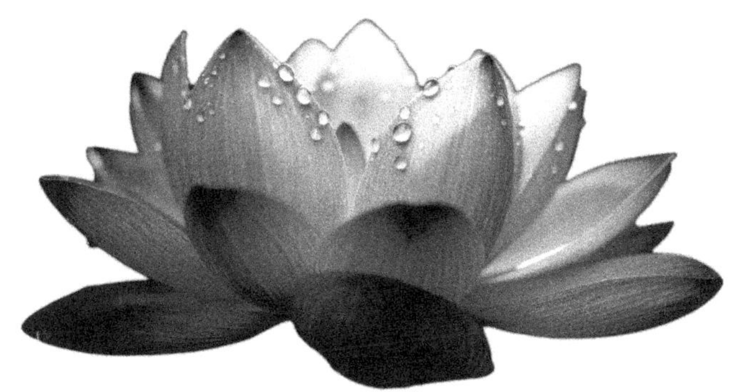

CATHERINE ALLARD

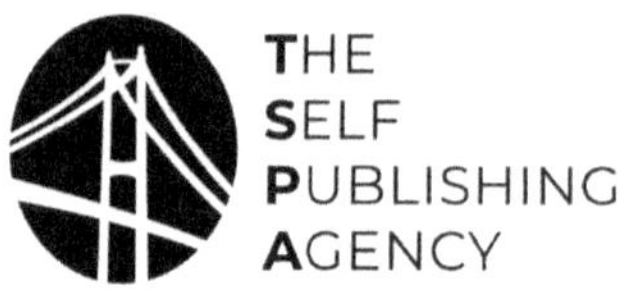

Catherine Allard
Becoming Comfortably Numb: A Memoir on Brain-Mending

Pineview Press
Copyright © 2024 by Catherine Allard
First Edition

Hardcover ISBN 978-1-7383973-1-0
Softcover ISBN 978-1-7383973-2-7
eBook ISBN 978-1-7383973-0-3

Book Design | Ashley Russell Designs
Editor | Kathie Lynas
Author Portrait Photography | Geneviève Maurice Photography
Publishing Management | TSPA The Self Publishing Agency, Inc.

For my husband and daughter

Your love and support make
everything possible

"To achieve the possible, we must attempt the impossible again and again."

Hermann Karl Hesse *(1877-1962)*
German-Swiss Poet, Novelist, Painter

Table of Contents

In Appreciation

I will never be able to name all the wonderful people who have helped me thrive over the years, but here's a list of the biggest clinical superstars. Despite many seemingly insurmountable challenges, their kindness, innovative ideas, expert treatments, therapies and advice allowed me to grasp, hang on to, and enjoy a full and happy life. This list reflects only their field of expertise at the time they treated me, and sadly, several of them have passed away. Also, there are others that I haven't named here (to protect their privacy) but I extend my deep gratitude to them as well.

Dr. Robert F. Nelson, Neurologist

Dr. C. Skinner, Neurology Resident

Dr. K.B. Mallya, Neurology Resident

Kathryn Eyre, Physiotherapist

Cynthia MacMillan, Massage Therapist

Lucie Hemstead, Neurological Physiotherapist

Andrea Plitz, Pelvic/Complex Issues Physiotherapist & Yogini

Dr. Sarah Vadeboncoeur, Naturopath

Monica Chappell, Yogini

Jennifer Spak, Osteopath & Massage Therapist

Dr. John Clifford, Physical Medicine & Rehabilitation

Sandi Millar, Registered Nurse

Céline Paris, Psychologist

Claudia Newman, Social Worker

Sandra Hobson, Occupational Therapist

Graham Curryer, Chiropodist

Nathalie Anglehart, Orthotist

Stefanie Goddyn, Chiropodist

Dr. P. Stys, Neurologist

Dr. M. Freedman, Neurologist

Dr. Ruth McPherson, Cardiologist

Dr. Barclay, Neurologist

Dr. H. C. De Meulemeester, Neurologist

Dr. L. Sitwell, Neurologist

Dr. A. McCormick, Pediatrics & Physical Medicine
& Rehabilitation

Ruth Thompson, Chiropodist

Dr. Jacques Brunet, Orthopaedic Surgeon

Dr. D. McCoubrey, Gynecological Surgeon

Dr. K. Baker, Urogynecological and Pelvic Reconstructive Surgeon

Dr. Luc Rochon, Gastrointestinologist

Dr. Benoit St-Jean, Surgeon

Dr. Louise Linney, Family Physician

Dr. Elie Skaff, Family Physician

Dr. McKeough, Medical Cannabis Counsellor

Dr. Lori Elliot, Medical Cannabis Counsellor

Dr. Mark Pogue, Optometrist

Neuro-ophthalmologists at The Eye Institute/University
of Ottawa

Catherine Bray, Occupational Therapist

Preface

Now a true senior citizen, at age 67, I feel like one of the luckiest women alive. I had my first stroke in 1984, at age 27, three months after delivering my precious baby girl.

Strokes, or "brain attacks," can arbitrarily crash down and suspend, scramble or kill a myriad of neural connections that your brain needs to direct not only movements of your body, but also your consciousness, perceptions, sensations and reasoning ability.

Strokes are a medical emergency. Plaque or a blood clot can either block off oxygen to a blood vessel in the brain, or a blood vessel can burst, and the bleeding can quickly suck the life out of you, even with immediate hospital intervention.

After the acute crisis, depending on the extent and areas of the brain that have been starved of oxygen and the type of immediate treatment you receive, physical and mental rehabilitation can often become a lifelong process.

Successful rehabilitation is hard work and depends on so many interdependent issues: the nature of your disabilities, how you and your body respond, how much useful clinical therapy you have access to, ongoing support from family, friends and the health care community, and your attitude. In the blink of an eye, you can die or become a vegetable, or else, every moment of your life can become one gigantic day-by-day struggle just to manage the basic activities of living.

But that's also why I feel so lucky.

Many die. Some people never regain the ability to walk or talk again. Discouragement and depression loom constantly.

But I got a second chance. And then, after another stroke six years later, a third chance at surviving.

I received tremendous rehabilitative care – the best that was available at that time. First, I had to get well enough to relearn how to walk, dress, clean and feed myself before I could learn how to feed, clean, clothe and carry the sweet, new, innocent life my husband and I had created. While in hospital full time and then as an outpatient, I missed out on my daughter's third to sixth months of life. In addition, the overwhelming heartache, and feelings of guilt and inadequacy robbed both my husband and me of many of the joys of first-time parenthood.

Even so, there was still so much joy, so much to live for. My daughter and I were still here on this Earth, and my husband and I could still live together and support each other under the same roof. We were in it together, in sickness and in health.

Then came yet another challenge for me and another long journey towards regaining my independence. In 1990, when my daughter was just starting Grade 2, I had another stroke. The second stroke was even more brutal than the first. It took several years for me to rebound, but I did, again, with incredible medical care and support around me.

Now life has truly come full circle, with my daughter becoming a mother to her own little girl. Becoming a grandmother has erased all but my most heart-breaking memories from 40 years ago, when I was lugging a custom-made, sandbag "baby" up and down the halls of Saint-Vincent Hospital to get enough strength and confidence to carry my own baby girl.

What follows is the story of my biggest struggles and greatest triumphs – from sobbing in a wheelchair all the way to climbing the Acropolis. It's also a story about how I have learned to manage my permanent limitations, on a day-to-day basis, and with the help of so many, regained a deeply satisfying communications career for longer than I ever expected. I hope to inspire realistic optimism for those living with or caring for anyone with disabilities or chronic health issues, all the more relevant today, with so many people suffering from neurological and other health after-effects due to COVID-19. With determination, we can always find small ways to break through and find happiness.

Today, there is so much more hope for stroke survivors, too. Now, teams of medical experts descend on the patient the moment they arrive and can perform immediate lifesaving treatments if appropriate. Clot-busting medical advances in acute stroke treatment that began in the mid-1990s are being refined to this day, resulting in miraculous total recoveries in certain patients with significant paralysis at the outset. Ottawa doctors recently became the first in the world to see inside our brain vessels using a flexible, microscopic camera that could lead to new treatments. The first trials for brain-bleed (or aneurism) treatments are also having amazing results, and the progress continues every day.

If you think you might be having a stroke, don't try to wait it out or go to bed hoping you'll feel better in the morning. Call an ambulance right away, so that you will be taken to the hospital and the medical professionals who can perform the best treatment available based on your symptoms.

Stroke is the number one cause of disability and loss of independence. Strokes can be very different for men and women, too. We should all familiarize ourselves with the most common signs of stroke and what to do, even if only to help those around us. Check out the Heart and Stroke Foundation of Canada | Home.

Never discount the potential impact of neuroplasticity – the brain's ability to "rewire" itself, and to adapt, heal and make new connections. Nor should you discount your own mind's potential to master your thoughts and habits, and learn how to do things "differently." Enough sleep, good nutrition, mindfulness, meditation, deep breathing, yoga and finding joy in simple things have all been scientifically proven to create synergies that can facilitate marked improvement.

Never forget how treatment innovations can turn the impossible into the possible.

Keep learning, whatever way you can.

Never forget the power of humour.

And (almost) Never Say Never. (Oops, I just did lol)

After 40 years, I still work hard every day to maintain and improve my changed abilities while still enjoying life, with the support of my devoted, nurturing husband (also known as Poppa Hen); my inspiring, sensible daughter and her beautiful family; our friends; and the healthcare community. I keep learning and adapting different ways to maintain what I've got left and keep it fun so I can Keep on Truckin'.

Finally, never take any of the opinions expressed here as medical advice. ALWAYS consult a trusted medical professional first before attempting anything new or different.

Round I

1

Half Gone, From Head to Toe

Whoopie! It's Saturday night!

On January 28, 1984, Jean-Pierre and I bundle our precious three-month-old daughter into her car seat and take a short drive over to some newish friends, Dave and Mimi Moores, who live close by, to play Trivial Pursuit for the first time. I'm feeling drained and struggling with a nasty migraine headache, but still really looking forward to enjoying a fun night out with lots of laughs.

As an extremely biased first-time mother, I know my sweet little baby girl (who will remain nameless, in respect of her privacy) is the best in the world. She eats well, is nearly always smiling and animated, naps well and has been sleeping through the night since she was merely six weeks old. We carefully bring our cherished infant inside Dave's house amongst jovial greetings, and then we attend to our "petite fille," still asleep in her portable car seat. We gently loosen off her snowsuit and station her in the darkened dining room to continue her sweet dreams. Then the four of us rustle up red wine and beer in the kitchen and lay out the boardgame on the big thick maple table, its benches gleaming. Let the games begin!

Soon after, we share a celebratory joint. I take one very light toke as sometimes, marijuana can help settle down one of my migraines.

The game is a hoot, and thanks also to the delectable glass of red wine, I feel very content, happily sitting there, despite feeling an insidious nausea rising from the brutal pounding in my head.

But then … *Aughhh! Geez! What the f … ?*

In a matter of seconds, a brutally cold, stinging wave suddenly clutches down through every fibre of my entire right side, from the top of my head, through half my nose, jaw and neck, down through my arm and torso, and further down, down, down through the arm and leg to the ends of my fingers and toes.

My entire right side has disappeared. I can see my arm, but it's no longer connected to me.

WTF???

Must try … just stand up … gotta try to walk around. Ohhh-myyy … tell me it's just asleep … my God … W-where is my right leg?

"Something's wrong!" I cry out.

In desperation, I start pushing to the left against Jean-Pierre, so I can slide across the bench and get out from against the wall. *I must stand up*, I tell myself. Looking confused, he quickly moves out of my way. I start to rise on my left leg but can't find my right arm to grasp the kitchen table.

I collapse onto the floor.

"Take me to the hospital," I say. I am terrified.

I don't know what's happening, but I know we are in deep, deep trouble.

Jean-Pierre looks dumbstruck. Somehow, he and Dave manage to carry me outside to the car and lay me down in the back seat.

Streetlights swoosh above me in the dark as JP floors it down Innes Road towards the General Hospital. Then I'm aware that he's struggling to get me out of the car and into a wheelchair. I am as cooperative as a rag doll.

I hear him insisting to one of the health professionals greeting us, "No! She has not just passed out from partying!"

Lesson #1: Always call an ambulance whenever you have a medical emergency. You'll be seen faster, and responders will be more prepared for you on arrival, especially with the continuing healthcare staff shortages worsened by the COVID-19 pandemic.

* * *

Later, I'm aware that I am lying on a stretcher in an extremely bright, high-tech private room. I am alone here for what seems like hours. At some point, I am told a call has been put in to a resident neurologist to come to the hospital to examine me.

Some time later, I hear a deep, calm voice calling my name in even, measured tones. I awaken to find a gravely serious, young Indian gentleman with dark brown eyes, chocolate skin and a rock-star mop of shiny black hair, staring at me intently.

"My name is Dr. Mallya," he says. "I am a neurological resident, and I will be examining you now."

He asks me lots of questions, encourages me to follow his wiggling fingers with each eye, and gently taps all over both sides of my body with a tiny reflex hammer. He looks directly into my eyes whenever he speaks, and although I am terrified, he is strangely calming.

"We are going to admit you," he finally pronounces. "And tomorrow we will be starting lots of tests."

Ah, what a relief … I don't know what's happening … but they'll figure it out …

He wasn't kidding about the volume of tests coming my way.

* * *

It's dark when I wake up again, but I can tell it's blisteringly sunny outside. *Oh, thank God, the blinds are closed. Head hurts so much. And feels so heavy. Like a cement ball. And the nausea …*

Hmmm, this is a private room. Good. My right side still feels completely numb, like it's not even there. But strangely, it also feels like it's on fire. The slightest movement of the bedsheets sends piercing electric shocks rippling through me. It even hurts to breathe, and it feels like I'm weighted down with lead.

Jesus! … just try not to move … just go back to sleep …

Later, a nurse comes in to check on me. She raises the back of the bed with the electric button to put me in a more upright position and shows me how to use the call button too. Then she positions the bedside tray across the bed and places a small plastic cup of something, either pudding or Jello, and a spoon, in front of me.

"Here, try to eat this," she says softly, smiling.

"What's happened?" I ask, hoping I don't sound too afraid.

"We're not sure just yet," she replied. "Tomorrow is Monday, so the doctors will start their rounds in the morning and order some tests. Your doctor is Dr. Nelson, who is Chief of Neurology. And the resident, Dr. Mallya, will be in to see you sometime later today."

Okay now, good. Dr. Mallya. I remember him. I trust him. That gives me some relief. I know he will figure out what's going on here.

After a while, I pick up the spoon with my left hand. I was right-handed, but now there's nothing but this horrible, heavy, stinging and burning blob of nothingness torturing my entire right side.

I notice that the little cup is a bit too far away from me. I can't seem to manoeuvre the spoon into the cup to drag it over, though. I put the spoon down to grab the cup. Everything hurts. I feel weepy, and my mind is racing with thoughts of catastrophe. *What the heck is wrong with me? I'm so young … so how could it be a stroke? How can something so simple be so difficult? How will I ever be able to take care of our darling baby daughter? How can JP manage everything right now, all by himself? He has to go to work. Oh dear … I am on maternity leave … and now feel like I'm a total failure as a mother … and how will I ever play piano? (I loved my music. I had achieved the level of Grade VIII Royal Conservatory and also had a wicked ear for Elton John, Supertramp and Deep Purple.) How will I use a pen … I am right-handed …*

I cry through gritted teeth.

Dammit! Every time I try to put the spoon in the cup, it starts sliding around.

*How can I f***ing eat this with one hand?*

Listlessly, I dip the spoon vertically and pull out a small blob. Sometimes it gets to my mouth before it falls.

I fear I will never be the same.

* * *

Dr. Mallya whisks in, all serious, objective and authoritative, save for his intensely sensitive eyes.

"How are you feeling today?" he asks quietly.

"Awful. It stings everywhere." I am trying to be brave.

He nods, and approaches. "I am going to check a few things out."

More eye tracking tests. More questions. More tapping, particularly on the leg. Very gentle.

Finished, he moves away from me, straightens up, and pauses a few moments, his eyes locking directly into mine.

"Raise your right hand off the bed," he says.

I am not expecting this. My eyes well up. "I can't …"

"Raise your right hand off the bed," he repeats, giving me no choice. I am taken aback by the quiet forcefulness of his command.

Where is my arm? I turn my head. Jeezus, ow ow … I look down, find the arm and Oh! Oh! Oh! Please stop these searing jolts everywhere … Why can't I tell where anything is?

His eyes are still boring into me. He must really think I can do this.

Lightning bolts scream everywhere. *Okay – I see my goddamn lifeless hand, but how do I raise it? Lift from the wrist first – now, from the elbow …*

This hurts like hell. I grit my teeth, take the deepest breath I can, and force, force and force …

Through the raging, burning icicles, I watch my hand. The wrist jerks up a few inches, lugging the arm up slightly from the elbow. It feels heavier than lead, but …

"Very good!" he exclaims, nodding once with a satisfied smile. *He knew I could do it.*

Immediately, my hand flumps back down onto the mattress. "Oh, God," I mutter. It burns so much.

"Tomorrow there will be a group of doctors making rounds and asking you a lot of questions," he announces. "Are you okay with that?"

"Sure. Will I see Dr. Nelson then?"

"Very soon," he assures me, "and I will see you again tomorrow."

Then, like a puff of smoke, he disappears.

Sometime later, JP visits. He cannot hide his grief and exhaustion. He has taken our baby, along with the playpen, to his mother, Thérèse. He tells me he went back to Dave's to retrieve her after I was admitted. I can't bear to think how awful it must have been for him to bring his little girl home all by himself, without her Mommy.

"At least I got you to show me how to prepare her bottles and use the washer and dryer a week ago," he says grimly, in a futile effort to bolster my spirits.

"Oh my … yes," I breathe, momentarily relieved, but the overshadowing grief made me feel like a complete failure as a mother. I had planned to nurse my little girl for three months, but decided to stop after two. I had been so tired; her birth had not been easy, and my energy had never returned.

My water had broken on Halloween night, during my treks back and forth to answer the door for the trick-or-treaters. The amniotic fluid was green instead of clear, so I called my obstetrician. He told me to eat a light meal and then get to the hospital, as there could be an increased risk of respiratory complications for the baby.

As soon as we arrived, a nurse slung a giant, heavy monitoring belt around my girth and told me not to move. I stayed there quietly for hours and hours.

Finally, when I was sufficiently dilated, I was given an epidural, but it fell out in the delivery room, and by then, it was too late to give me another one.

"There are signs of fetal distress now," my obstetrician said tersely, after 26 hours of labour. "We have to get the baby out. It's time for a Cesarean."

But I refused his directions and made a deal with the devil.

"Please, just let me push once more," I begged. He acquiesced with reluctance, and before he could change his mind, I took the deepest breath I could, gritted my teeth and bore down, down, down … something started to give …

"Okay … there's the head … it's a girl!"

I smiled, completely spent. I heard my daughter cry, which filled my heart, and noticed a nurse carrying a small bundle towards the scale. This was reassuring, but there seemed to be too much activity around me. And very little talking.

"She's beautiful," said Jean-Pierre, grasping my hand. Then I just closed my eyes and let go, until a nurse carefully positioned our new bundle of joy by my side.

"Seven pounds, 11 ounces," she said kindly. That was a good weight.

Still, she seemed so tiny, so pale, and so serious. It had been a tough go for her too. My last big defiant push ended with a huge cervical tear as she came into the world. I wish I'd complied with my obstetrician's advice to have a Cesarean.

2

Delayed Diagnosis

Early Monday morning, the neurology ward at the Ottawa General was abuzz. As Dr. Mallya had warned, a hive of six white coats suddenly swarmed in and landed around my bedside. Their keen, intensely interested expressions could not allay their quiet concern that they weren't quite sure what they were looking at. There were many introductions, many, many questions, and many tests both initially and in the days after, before I would learn they had zeroed in on two possible diagnoses. This was just the bare beginning.

"Look straight ahead. Now tell me when you can see my fingers coming from the left. Good, and now from the right." My right eye couldn't see the fingers until they were almost directly in front of me. That explained why everyone coming into the room from my right surprised me; I had lost peripheral vision on my right side.

They loved to tap my arms and legs with a little hammer, run a little metal wand against the bottoms of both feet, and then poke me all over.

"Can you tell me exactly where I am touching you?" No, I could not. On my right side, I had only a vague sense of where the horrific burning increased.

"What is your family history of heart attacks and stroke?"

"Well, I know my Grandmother had her first heart attack at 48 and died at 69, and my Mother has a congenital heart defect."

"Was that your Grandmother on your Mom's side of the family?"

"Yes. I think there might have been a few others too. I'll ask my Mom to send me more details."

"What about multiple sclerosis?"

"Not that I know of."

"Does your face get red when you run?"

"Yes, pretty often."

"Did you take the pill?"

"Yes."

"Do you smoke?"

"Yes, although I had cut down to under 10 a day when I was expecting."

In 1984, you could still smoke at the office. Hard to believe nowadays. Heck, smoking was even allowed inside the Ottawa General Hospital at that time. A few days later, when another random group of white coats swarmed in, they could not hide their alarm when they caught me tapping my cigarette ashes into a tiny medicine cup. I shrank back with shame, quickly butting out the evil "fag." It was one of the last cigarettes I ever smoked.

A few days passed before we actually met Dr. Nelson, the Chief of Neurology. Apparently he was a very busy man.

Dr. Skinner, the lead resident, usually made an appearance every day. He wore roundish wire glasses on his kind, pale, quietly cheerful face. With his short, wavy blond hair, he appeared to be roughly the same age as JP and me.

"I think I have some idea what you two are going through right now," he said softly, the first time we met. "My wife and I have a baby girl at home too, and she's the same age as your daughter."

The first week in hospital was a miserable blur of testing.

Near the end of that week, Dr. Mallya appeared, gingerly perched himself on the end corner of my bed, and took a moment or two before making eye contact with me. He had never acted this way before.

"Given your young age," he began, "You've had either a "cerebrovascular accident" or a stroke, as it's more often called, and in your case, caused by a blood clot – or there is also a possibility it could be the onset of multiple sclerosis, or MS."

"MS?" I mouthed, flabbergasted. He nodded, diverting his eyes.

"Sometimes when young people experience their first MS attack, it can mimic a stroke. We need to get a clear diagnosis before we can start treatment, because the two conditions are so different."

My throat clenched with despair.

"Any questions?"

I shook my head. "No, just do whatever you have to do …" And with a grateful nod, he vanished.

Of the two possible grave diagnoses, I prayed that it was a stroke, because there was so much more hope for improvement. I had to have hope that one day I would get well enough to care for my daughter and love my hubby the way he deserved to be loved. From the little I already knew about MS, there was no cure – it was an eventual death sentence.

Dr. Nelson, the Chief of Neurology, had a special interest in MS. I had CAT scans to map brain damage, Doppler (echo) scans to trace the blood flow of the arteries in my neck, echocardiograms to check out my heart, and blood pressure monitoring at least twice a day, plus a gallon of blood tests and visual tests. In the latter category I had a test conducted in a tiny chamber, where my pounding head was hooked up to electrodes, and I had to stare at a screen of tiny, dizzying black-and-white squares shifting back and forth, side to side, and up and down for what seemed like hours.

A speech pathologist determined I didn't appear to have aphasia, or any issues with speaking or communicating. This was great news, because with stroke, when the right side is affected, speech can often suffer. And communications was my career. I had been enjoying burgeoning responsibilities in advertising and communications in a hectic environment at Export Development Corporation. *Oh Good God … what am I going to do about that?*

A physiotherapist visited me early on to test my range of

motion and manipulate my right arm and leg. She brought weird rulers and geometric measurement discs to compare functionality on both sides.

The next morning, she produced a brown paper bag filled with various everyday items – a watch, a comb, a rubber ball, a spoon – and placed the bag close to my right hand.

"Please place your right hand in the bag, and without looking, try to find the watch," she said.

I got my brain to convince the lead-weighted right hand to inch over and into the bag, but I couldn't even tell if my fingers were moving, let alone where. Nothing but stinging, everywhere.

"It's useless," I lamented, near tears, dismissing the useless hand.

She said that I was making quick progress in regaining physical strength and functioning, even though I had very little sensation of what limb she was touching or what I was moving on my right side without watching myself do it. The inability to identify an object by active touch in the absence of vision is known as "astereognosis."

I felt destroyed. I was right-handed. How was I going to be able to pick up a pen, let alone write with one? How was I going to be able to hold or carry my little papoose? Or take care of her?

⋆ ⋆ ⋆

After about five days, Dr. Mallya came in, looking particularly grave. "Good morning," he said. "So far, all the tests we have conducted have been inconclusive."

"Oh, crap. So now what?"

"Well, we think you need to have a cerebral angiogram," he

said softly. "That is the only way to confirm whether you have had a stroke, by finding a blood clot in your brain. And if it is a blood clot, then you'll need to start being treated with anticoagulants as soon as possible."

"That sounds pretty serious."

He nodded. "Yes, it is. We will insert an IV and run some dye through your brain, and that will tell us if there is a clot. However, this kind of test is considered invasive, as there is always a very small risk of complications," he said.

"Complications? Like what?"

He held his gaze. "Well, on very rare occasions, a clot could move inside the brain and cause more damage," he explained. "But in your case, we all agree the need to know definitely outweighs the risk. We will also need you to sign a permission form before we can proceed."

He waited a moment. "Do you think you're okay with this?"

"Well … if you think it's necessary," I murmured, feeling surprise and unexpected dread in the realization that he was trying to persuade me to take a risk. I understood what he was telling me and I trusted him, but he could tell I was petrified.

"Don't worry," he assured me. "I will be there during the test to keep an eye on everything. Are we okay then?"

My nod brought about a tiny smile from him. "Very good. Within the next hour, someone should be coming to bring you over for prep and to have you sign the form. I'm not certain in what order that will happen though."

"Okay."

He nodded once, then whirled away. "See you later," he called from the hallway.

⁕ ⁕ ⁕

Two porters arrived first. They nimbly transferred me from the bed onto a stretcher. The ride seemed endless. Finally, we passed through some heavy swinging doors and entered a huge, brightly lit forum with a glassed-in viewing gallery high up near the ceiling, at the top of a flight of stairs. The glaring lights made my head pound, and I had to close my blinded eyes to slits in order to see anything. I recognized Dr. Skinner and others among a small assembly of gawking white coats while I was being hooked up to IVs, tubes and alien machines by a couple more white coats. Panic rose in my throat. Was I a lab rat or something? What's going to happen to me? What if there's a clot, and it travels?

And where is Dr. Mallya?

Just then, a door opened at the bottom of the stairs, and he appeared. He looked my way, and gave me a slight nod before gliding upstairs toward his colleagues. I felt a bit calmer now. The Resident Magician had arrived, as promised.

A female voice came to me from the upper left now. "Mrs. Allard?" Someone was holding a clipboard and placing a pen in my left hand. "Would you please sign the permission form right here?"

The pen flailed somewhere on the paper. I felt strangely like I was observing myself. *Yes, of course. You now have permission to kill me. Or turn me into a vegetable …*

"Thank you," the soft voice said. A masked face made earnest eye contact with me. "We are just about ready to get started. Now even though you have been sedated, you may still feel some discomfort during the procedure. Any questions?"

I shook my head. *No, just get this over with …*

"Alright. Here we go." I took a deep breath. A switch flicked, followed by high-pitched thrumming.

And suffocating agony.

Overwhelming heat rushed through my skull. Every blood vessel in my head felt like it was on fire. Ready to explode. Even worse, nauseating, acrid burning rubber seared my nostrils and the back of my mouth, growing worse and worse every nanosecond … on … and on … and on … I could not breathe or swallow, and I prayed not to choke, vomit or have my head explode …

Finally, mercifully, the whining subsided. My lead-weighted head felt like a quivering mass of wet cement. I inhaled a ragged breath, relieved that I could breathe again. It remains to this day the most horrifying hospital procedure I have ever experienced.

"We're all done now, Cathy. You did really well."

Eyes half closed, I did not bother to acknowledge anyone as they detached me from the equipment. I was in a fugue – totally spent, and simply relieved to have survived this brief but severe bout of horror.

"We're going to bring you back to your room now, and we'll know the results very soon."

The rest of the day was a complete blank, except for a brief visit from JP. He looked gobsmacked. All we could think about was getting the diagnosis. I don't even remember who was taking care of our child.

* * *

The next morning, shortly after the cursed left-handed struggle to eat my f***ing breakfast, Dr. Mallya appeared, looking more gentle than usual.

"Good morning. How are you feeling?"

I shrugged. "Well, much better than yesterday, at least. Any results from the test?"

"Yes," he said, with a dutiful nod. "We found a blood clot. You have had a stroke."

He stood silently, politely observing me while I processed this. My first reaction was relief for finally knowing what I was dealing with. And secondly, relief that it was not multiple sclerosis, a degenerative neurological disease, for which there is no cure.

"You are very young to have had a stroke," he told me. "But that also means you will recover much faster than someone in, say, their sixties."

Hmm. I supposed it was good that I would become a fierce competitor among the ranks of the aged, even though I wasn't able to take care of my daughter.

His positivity bolstered me, though. "Okay, please raise your right arm as high as you can."

With gritted teeth, and through the bitter stinging, my eyes found what looked like my arm and helped my brain figure out how to coax what felt like a heavy lump of lead to obey almost automatically this time, and I was able to raise it above my shoulder before it flopped down again.

"See? Your range of motion has improved a great deal."

"Okay … but … how come there is so much stinging every-where on my right side?"

"Well, there may be several reasons," he said quietly. "First of all, it's still very early. Your brain is in shock. And every stroke is different. It depends on which areas of the brain are damaged, to what extent, and how it affects each individual. In your case, we think the blood clot has affected your thal-amus, which is the part of the brain that controls your sensations – including touch, eyesight and hearing."

"Oh. Okay." *Well at least I'm not completely blind, and I can still hear, but boy … those horrible electric shocks all over my right side … with every move I make …*

"Dr. Nelson will come and see you later today to discuss this with you in more detail," he said quickly. "But the first thing we must do right away is dissolve the blood clot. We'll be putting you on heparin intravenously. Heparin is an anti-coagulant, and we will be testing your blood daily, until we are satisfied that it's under control."

"Okay, that sounds good."

He nodded respectfully. "In the meantime, you will con-tinue to receive physiotherapy, and a few other tests perhaps, but nothing major like yesterday. And once you're on the IV," he added, "we can get you out of bed, and you can start walking again."

That is very good news. I smiled.

"I should also mention that you have a reduction in the

peripheral visual field in your right eye; it's known as a field cut."

"Ah, so that's why I keep getting surprised when people just seem to appear in front of me from my right side."

"That would make sense, yes," he concurred. "Your hearing in your right ear may have also been affected."

Geez. This is a lot to take in.

"It is quite fortunate though that your speech does not appear to be affected," he told me. "Strokes affecting the right side can often cause speech and communication problems."

For the first time, I felt extremely lucky because, as I've mentioned, communications was my gig.

"Any idea why this happened?" I dared to ask.

His face fell. "We can't really say for sure at this point. You mentioned there was a family history?"

"Yes. My mother is supposed to be putting a list together and will mail it to me from Vancouver. I will give it to you as soon as I get it."

"Yes, that would be good to know. Any other questions?"

(Other than a million and one?) I shook my head.

"Alright then, you'll be put on the heparin IV very shortly, and Dr. Nelson will see you soon," he said with a nod before sweeping out of the room. I was learning that residents had their plates heavily loaded.

* * *

With the heparin IV inserted into my right arm, the burning intensified at the entrance point, with lightning bolts continually assaulting my arm whenever I inadvertently pulled on the tubing without realizing it. Neither did I fully appreciate that I was now learning all sorts of different ways to get used to my new reality. All I knew was that it hurt like hell all the time, and it was so exhausting having no escape from it. I felt very sorry for myself.

The authoritative Dr. Nelson made his eventual appearance, with the cheerful Dr. Skinner in tow. Slight in stature with a pale, dour face, the Neurology Chief's eyes seemed hooded and devoid of emotion under his large, thick-lensed glasses. He was a man of few words – quietly polite, but intimidating. He said far less than Dr. Mallya, except that there didn't appear to be anything wrong with my heart, and that he wanted to do a few more tests, particularly vision tests, to completely rule out MS.

"MS? I thought it was a stroke."

"Yes, it was. But since you are so young and you are already in the hospital, we just want to completely rule out MS because your experience was quite similar to what happens with early-onset MS patients."

Oh wow. Just when I thought we had a clear diagnosis …

Dr. Nelson also mentioned that after a stroke, the greatest recovery happens in the first six months, and then up to approximately two years after that. (It should be noted that in 1984, there was no concept of "neuroplasticity" – the idea that after brain damage, the brain can in fact continue to find new neurons and pathways to facilitate small and continued improvements, long after two years. Usually, these tiny progressions can happen only after diligent focus and practice, and with the right kind of stimulation. But after

40-some years, I can certainly attest to the validity of neuroplasticity.)

While I have indeed aged in many ways, I continue to find new ways to perceive things through the pins and needles. For example, I can now clumsily grasp onto a set of keys in my right pocket because I can determine when the largest car key is digging into my palm, since metal stings more than anything else, and the larger the sting, the better. It's like finding your own best way, given your situation, to do something differently, and then building on that synergy to get even better at it. However, I still constantly misplace things I pick up with my right hand, because when I'm not looking at it, my brain doesn't register that it's there, and I forget I'm holding onto something.

"You are otherwise strong and healthy too, so you should do very well," Dr. Nelson added.

No one was saying I would make a full recovery, though, and I didn't need to ask. All that ran through my mind was dread about how, when or if I would ever be able to cradle and carry my darling baby girl again, let alone be a good enough mother to her. That was a huge motivation, though – I could not even think of giving up.

* * *

The next morning, a physiotherapist appeared with a very tall walker. It had no wheels. My eyes widened with fearful anticipation.

"Good morning, Cathy! We've got the go-ahead to get you up and about."

I stared at her blankly. I had absolutely no idea what to do.

"We're going to start very, very slowly," she said kindly, as if reading my mind. "Having been in bed for a week, all your muscles are going to feel very stiff and much weaker. Today, we'll probably just get you used to sitting on the edge of the bed, and maybe work on safely transferring from the bed to the walker. Sound good?"

"Yes, bring it on."

She reached under the bed for a switch and lowered the bed as close to the floor as possible.

"Now don't worry about the IV pole for now. It's got wheels and I will manage that for you. Is the back of your bed completely upright, or can you raise yourself a bit more?"

There was an electronic lever on my left side that I could operate quite easily by now, so I tilted the back of the bed up to the max.

The physiotherapist gently removed the sheets from my legs. While the room wasn't cold, the fresh air hit my right leg like a raging mass of pinpricks. I shrank back, grimacing.

"Stinging?"

"Mm-hmm."

"Take some deep breaths, and try to relax. Easy for me to say, right?"

I smiled grimly. "Whenever you're ready, bend your knees a little. Good. Now try to pivot at the waist and move your lower legs over the edge of the bed. I'll be spotting you, so don't worry about losing your balance. At this point, all I want you to do is sit up straight at the edge of the bed, okay?"

I nodded. For a couple of days now, while lying down, we had already been practising sliding the soles of my feet towards me along the mattress to bend my knees, then moving them back and forth like windshield wipers.

"Now you may feel dizzy or light-headed once you're sitting up, but don't worry; that's normal. And don't forget that you've always got your left hand to ground you if you need it. But try to avoid relying on it. Focus on keeping your core strong." She had the IV pole in her hand with the walker close by and moved in closer. "Ready?"

I nodded and got started. I had already figured out that guiding my weakened right leg with the stronger left one helped ground me. My physio guide had her fingers touching my shoulders to help steady my upper body. Moving the right leg was like pushing a heavy lead beam against a brick wall. Scream-worthy sparks flew everywhere, but slowly, my legs were moving.

"Good! Now get ready to lean forward, and turn at the waist ..."

Well now, I am actually sitting at the edge of the bed! I hear "very good!" in the background, but dammit ... masses of razor blades everywhere ... my neck and cheek and my arm and leg are so heavy, like lead weights ... and I am SO tired ... my head is spinning ... everything hurts ... hurts way too much ...

I close my eyes and suck in a ragged breath.

"A bit dizzy?"

"Yeah, and it stings really bad too. Even half my butt's on fire," I joked.

"That's okay, Cathy, you're doing great. Take all the time you need." She positioned the walker so that the high, rounded handlebars were about a six-inch reach away. "Do you feel like continuing?"

"You bet, now that I'm up."

"Now, whenever you feel ready, grasp and hold on to the bars with both hands, and make sure your right hand is secure. This walker will not move; it has no wheels. For now, we're just going to focus on holding on to it before we get you on your feet, all right?"

I nodded, and reached toward the bars. I gazed at my stinging right stump of a hand and found myself watching its fingers, willing them to curl themselves around the metal bar. But as soon as they made contact, my hand jerked back involuntarily, as if it had just plunked down on a hunk of dry ice.

"Ow!" I yelped. "So cold!" I noticed my therapist's surprised expression. I wish I could remember her name. She was so kind.

Now that I knew what to expect, I repositioned the hand and did my best to hold fast. The heavy arm was quick to weaken and seize up from the strain. I was told this was because my stroke had resulted in high spasticity, causing choppy, irregular movements on my right side. I dropped my arms to my sides for a moment.

"Just taking a little breather."

"No worries, Cathy. Next time you grab the bars, you can try putting your feet down on the floor and standing up. I'll be right next to you. And that'll be all we're going to do today."

I looked down. My feet were just a few inches off the floor, but I was terrified I would collapse. I had no idea where among the stinging mass of numbness that thing that was supposed to be my right foot was, unless I continually stared down at it. But the physiotherapist was right next to me, with her steady hand behind my back, reassuring me that she could guide me back to the bed if necessary.

"Okay, I'm ready."

"Again, make sure your fingers are curled around the handles."

Ew! Stingies … "Now inch forward – touch down with your left toes first – good. Now, I'm watching your rightie, so go ahead, put it down on the floor, and then push up … "

OHMYGODSHIT HORRID SPARKS EVERYWHERE … UGH … OK … THERE'S MY LEG … AND MY FOOT … I SEE THEM … BUT THEY JUST BURN BURN, BURN …

"Excellent! You're standing!"

After a few seconds, I closed my eyes and curled back down onto the bed, completely spent. I wanted to cry.

"It feels so awful."

"It will get easier, Cathy. You did really well," my physiotherapist said, smiling calmly. "And good news – your husband will be bringing in your running shoes tonight. So tomorrow, I will show you an easy way to tie your shoelaces with one hand, and then we can try taking a few steps."

Well at least that gives me something to look forward to. It's literally baby steps now …

At that moment, I felt just as helpless as my darling baby girl.

"And the single-hand lacing is just a temporary measure. I'm sure you'll be tying them with both hands before you leave here."

I nodded weakly. *So tired … can't compute …*

"Here, let me help you get settled," she said, guiding my legs back on the mattress, and covering me.

"Again, well done Cathy. See you tomorrow."

I murmured thanks and curled up into a fetal position on my

left side. The stupid IV was pulling at me somewhere on my arm, but I didn't care. If I yanked it out, someone could just come in and reconnect it, goddammit. I buzzed the nurse for more pain meds. Surely by now it had been four hours since the last dose. The pain overwhelmed me, wave after wave. All I could do was try not to drown in my silent tears.

⁎ ⁎ ⁎

JP had taken the first week off work after my stroke, mostly to overcome the shock and organize himself as Poppa Hen, as I eventually came to call him. Luckily, he had asked me to show him how to make formula, sanitize bottles and run the washer and dryer less than two weeks before I abandoned them – talk about serendipity!

When he came to visit me in the evenings during visiting hours, either his mother, Thérèse, would look after our bundle of joy, or our close friend, Gail Campeau – a high school girlfriend and now mother of four children with her husband Jean – generously pitched in during the first couple of weeks.

That night, JP arrived with my running shoes in one hand, and in the other, our barely three-month old baby girl, fast asleep in her portable car seat/baby carrier. I burst into tears. It was the first time I'd seen her since the night our lives changed forever. Seeing them together like that broke my heart; he looked so exhausted and grief-stricken, and she was so tiny and helpless.

"Oh … my little sweetie," I choked, as JP set down the carrier at the end of the bed and started unbuckling her. "I … I'm so sorry for leaving you and Papa."

He gently lifted her up, cradled her in his arms and brought her over to me, his nervous face tight. "How do you want to do this?"

"I don't know!" I sobbed. "I can't even hold her."

"Here," he said, gently tucking her in between me and my left arm. "You two can just stay like that for a little while, okay?"

Her warm, soft face nestled against mine, and the sweet sensation of her random movements momentarily comforted me. She smelled so clean and fresh in her fuzzy, white terry sleeper. She oozed contentment, calmly taking in everything around her. But when her huge wide eyes met mine, I was again overcome with grief and guilt because I was failing her and Jean-Pierre. I nestled my lips against her cheek, trying to calm myself, but I couldn't suppress my rising agitation. I couldn't stop crying. I was her mother, but I wasn't. I couldn't BE her Mom. Heck, I couldn't even hold her! How would I ever be able to look after her?

"Please," I hiccupped, through sobs. "Just take her … please. I can't – she can't be here with me and all this negative energy … I'm just … not ready."

Jean-Pierre looked like I had just thrust a dagger into his heart. "What's wrong?"

"Oh … everything … they got me out of bed today and had me stand up, holding onto a walker … it was so awful … "

He frowned through his tender focus to retrieve our little darling and carefully positioned her in his arms. "But that's great, isn't it? You actually stood up?"

"Yes, but there was so much burning, all the time … and I was so dizzy … and I can't even tell where my foot is when it's on the floor. It's just a dead piece of meat with pins and needles, pins and needles … and every move makes me so exhausted."

"Well, maybe it'll go a bit easier tomorrow?" he peeped, his voice so small. He was trying to encourage me, but he couldn't hide his despair.

"I sure hope so," I sighed. "I'm so sorry … "

"Don't say that, hon. I brought your shoes for tomorrow, like they told me. I put them in your closet."

"Oh … thanks … " I whimpered. "Th-they say I'm young … and if I work hard … I'll improve quickly." I found it hard to look at them through my tears. I felt so defeated.

We exchanged a few more strained words as JP hurriedly bundled our tiny sweet pea back into her snowsuit and into her carrier. He looked like he was barely holding it together himself, trying not to break down in front of me.

"I love you," he whispered. He leaned over our baby and kissed my forehead. "I'll see you tomorrow, and I can't wait to hear about your first steps."

"Me too, and I p-promise to try my best … "

* * *

The next morning my physiotherapist showed up with the walker right after the docs had finished their morning rounds.

"Good morning. Are your running shoes in your closet?"

"Yup. JP brought them last night."

"Great." She retrieved them, and began to pull out the laces on each shoe. "Before we get started, I'm going to show you how to tie your shoelaces with one hand. Again, I don't think you'll need to do this for very long, but at least it will give you more independence."

She demonstrated the technique for me a few times. "It looks sort of funny, with only half a loop, but it does the job. Want to try it?"

"Yeah, sure."

With a soft smile, she opened up the left shoe wide and gave it to me. "Try putting it on by yourself, and don't worry about messing up the bed."

Gritting my teeth, I leaned forward, willing myself to shut out the raging on my right side. I found it surprisingly easy to get the shoe onto my foot with one hand, since I was in bed and didn't have to think about falling or losing my balance. And shock of shocks, I did the half loop on the first attempt!

"Whoo hoo!"

"Fantastic! Think you're up to try the right shoe?"

"Sure! I'm on a roll, right?"

She opened up the shoe as wide as she could. "Here you go."

"OH! That's bad!"

Reaching over with my left hand towards my right foot sent screaming shocks across my chest and waist, and my right arm jerked, pulling on the IV line. Carefully, I sat back for a moment and took a couple of deep breaths.

"That was very unpleasant."

"Take all the time you need."

Again, I gritted my teeth and fumbled to get the shoe over the nasty stinging stump. I was grinding; the foot defied my wishes until I figured out how to open up the shoe wide enough to force the foot inside.

I fell back on the bed, exhausted.

"Good job!"

"You mean good half-job, " I corrected, almost panting from the exertion. "Still need to do it up."

"You'll get there."

I didn't want to take too long, though. If I thought about the pins and needles too much, I wouldn't want to move again. Besides, now I knew I could tie my shoe, so I took another deep breath and held it until the shoe was tied. It was much more onerous than the left one though because of the increased distance and angle I had to move my torso. (As an aside, it didn't take my dentist long to insist that I wear a mouthguard at bedtime to protect what was left of my teeth, after I had ground down my once-pointed incisors to flat lines. Chronic pain and clenched, grinding teeth often share a vicious symbiosis.)

I heard my physiotherapist clapping. "You did it!"

I felt better and couldn't help but smile. "I guess now you're gonna force me to haul myself out of bed and start walking."

"Yup. Whenever you're ready."

I knew I could make myself stand up. I had done it yesterday, and now today, I had put shoes on my feet. All by myself. So this time, the process of wiggling myself over to the edge of my bed, grasping the walker and pushing myself up to stand was much easier. I was determined to succeed.

"Wow! Very good!"

I continued to smile between ragged breaths. I was standing up!

"Now, as you're about to take your first half a step, try to lift the walker just above your feet, and then put it down just a little bit forward, before you place your foot on the floor. It's probably going to be a pretty clumsy process, but your safety right now is most important. Whenever you're ready … "

I looked down at the burning masses that used to be my right hand and foot. They were already trembling with weakness, weighted down, leaden. How long could I stay standing like this and support my weight? And how could I make my right arm rise along with the left to lift the walker?

I managed to raise the walker, mostly from the left side, but then I couldn't figure out where I was. I was lost inside it; I had no control of it, and it kept jerking away from me to the left while going nowhere at the same time. I was rewarded with what was probably a sliding half step, but then the walker locked on me, as it was meant to, stopping me from falling.

"Crap!"

All I could do was just hang on with intensity and stay upright through all the burning pins and needles. I had hardly any idea where I was or how I was positioned.

"That was great! Now take a little break; take a few breaths and look at how you're positioned."

"This walker is not very friendly," I spat. "The handlebars are too high."

"Yes, I know, but it's all we have right now, and the bars can't be adjusted," she said softly. "It really is the safest way for you to get started, and I don't think you'll need to use it for very long. So, let's try taking another step now … raise the walker, and lead with your right foot this time."

I looked down to watch myself lift and push my right foot forward while trying to raise the *(stupid mule)* walker in sync with my step. Again I got slammed to a halt. More godforsaken sparks. The fatigue was intense, but I had taken my first step on my affected side.

"Hurray!" My therapist's eyes sparkled with delight. "Another?"

I nodded and clumsily pressed on. I think I managed three more herky-jerky steps before I had to beg off. My kind physio somehow helped me back to the bed safely and removed my shoes for me. Baby steps. Well, at least now I could say I was ahead of my daughter.

"That was incredible work today, Cathy. I'll see you tomorrow."

I sank back into a quasi-comatose state, absolutely blown away by all the personal attention I was getting, and by how all these dedicated healthcare professionals, complete strangers to me, were working so hard trying to help me heal.

* * *

JP came in after supper. His eyes looked less grave. I could tell he had some big news.

"What's up?"

"Gloucester Family Day Care set up an appointment for me to interview a caregiver today, and it went really well," he said.

"Oh, that's wonderful, hon. What a relief!"

"I'll say," he said softly. "Three months old is the youngest age they'll accept, so yes, thank goodness."

We had applied to our neighbourhood childcare service before

I went on maternity leave from Export Development Corporation (a federal crown corporation now known as Export Development Canada or EDC), assuming that I would go back to work after my six months off. I was a Type-A aspiring career girl, a Carleton University School of Journalism drop-out who had worked her way up from a secretarial position to the professional ranks as a junior marketing officer.

"The caregiver's name is Debra Laxton," JP continued. "She has two little girls of her own, Kessa and Kyla, and she's also looking after a little boy named David. She seems very nice; she's quite soft-spoken but also firm with her kids."

"Oh. Wow. Does she live close to us?"

"Yeah. She's in Pineview too, just a couple of blocks away. Everyone seemed very happy, and our girl could start going there this coming Monday."

"Wow. Everything's happening so fast," I murmured. "It's so weird that I haven't even met the person who's going to be taking care of our daughter."

* * *

The next evening, Jean-Pierre brought me an envelope. It was the letter from my mom, listing her mother's 12 brothers and sisters, their various ailments, and how they died.

Every sibling died from cardiovascular issues, and three suffered their first incident before the age of 50.

The information shocked me so much that I couldn't comprehend how I hadn't known or been told beforehand.

This was the first I'd heard of the magnitude of the genetic cardiovascular "weakness" on my mother's side. I knew my Granny Driedger had her first heart attack at 48 and died of a stroke at 69. Back then though, nobody talked about their health problems. They were usually withheld as a dirty secret – a sign of personal inadequacy.

The next morning, Dr. Mallya floated in, looking cheerful. I didn't smile back though. I was just waiting to give him my mother's cursed genealogy letter.

"Good morning," he said.

I just nodded. He looked surprised by my glumness.

"So, I understand you're walking now," he said. "That's excellent."

"Oh. Yeah." I looked down at the letter on the bed beside me. His eyes followed. "That's my family history you asked about."

"Oh yes, thank you." He picked up the letter; his long dark fingers nimbly unfolding it. Almost immediately, his eyes widened, then darkened and held intensely for a good minute, as he reviewed the poorly-typed list.

"This is very significant," he said, after a few moments. "May I make a photocopy of this?"

"Of course. I had no idea about the extensiveness of my family history," I said. "And I smoked cigarettes and took the pill … "

He nodded, acknowledging my distress, but still, he looked encouraging. "Well, I have some other news for you that's a bit better."

"Oh?"

"Yes. I've been told that once the heparin has done its job thinning your blood, and you get a bit stronger, you will be transferred to the Rehabilitation Centre."

"Oh, that IS good news," I said, without even thinking. Subconsciously, I knew that I was going to need a great deal of help to figure out how to do things differently, since I had no idea how I would ever be able to do things the same way I did before. I sensed it would probably take a long time, too.

In the meantime, there was still lots of hard work to do. I ended up staying in acute care at the General Hospital for three weeks before changing institutions.

* * *

Every morning, the medical team would come in and poke me here and prod me there, so they could assess how my mobility, visual and sensation issues were coming back. Because it was a teaching hospital, the younger residents usually asked me a myriad of questions. Perhaps I was an interesting anomaly for them. I was not their typical stroke patient in terms of declining health or increased age, so they were particularly motivated to try to figure out the "how and why" it happened. Also, at 27 years old with an infant, the odds for successful rehabilitation were better for me than for most. The prospects for me relearning how to live independently and care for others were promising.

I actually looked forward to their visits. I too had a lot of questions for them, so it was very illuminating. Prior to having the stroke, I really never understood what it meant to have one. The biggest thing I learned is that every stroke is different – depending on whether it's a blood clot or a blood vessel bleed (known as an aneurism), what side and what parts of the brain are affected, and to what degree. And even then, it would not be fair to generalize as to how that damage will manifest or be expressed in the individual, or how well they will recover. And at that point, I really had no idea how I would move forward.

* * *

I was allowed pain meds every four hours, but it was never enough.

At the start of the week during which I was to be transferred to rehabilitation therapy, Dr. Mallya came in looking a little frazzled.

"So … how are you doing this morning?"

"Getting anxious to go to the Rehab Centre. Any idea when that's going to be?"

He looked down as if searching for the right words. "Umm, definitely towards the end of the week," he said. "Only you won't be going to the Rehabilitation Centre after all. You have a spot confirmed at Saint-Vincent Hospital, instead."

My initial reaction was disappointment. The Rehab Centre had such a stellar reputation. I had lived in Ottawa since 1967 and had never once heard of Saint-Vincent Hospital.

"It's primarily a chronic care hospital," he continued, "but they have an excellent stroke rehabilitation ward on their main floor. It will be more appropriate for you there, given your issues. The Rehabilitation Centre is for more complex cases like traumatic head injuries or amputations, where the recovery process is much longer than yours will be."

"Oh. Well I guess that's good, then."

"Yes," he declared. "It's very good."

* * *

Jean-Pierre hit the roof when I told him that evening.

"Saint-Vincent's? Shit!! You can't go there! That place is run by nuns and people stay there till they croak! That's where you go when your condition can't be managed at home!"

"But Dr. Mallya told me they also have a really good stroke rehab program there."

"I don't care! This is ridiculous! I'm calling Dr. Nelson tomorrow!"

As the week progressed, Friday was finally declared the transfer day. I can't remember if JP actually called Dr. Nelson, but I was still heading to Saint-Vincent's.

I was terrified because I had no idea what to expect. I was also upset because I would be forced to deal with a whole new group of healthcare professionals. I'd already had no choice but to completely open myself up to endure so much intimate poking, prodding, procedures, tests and questions by the wonderful team at the Ottawa General Hospital, and I had developed so much trust and respect for them and all their efforts to help me. Particularly Dr. Mallya. I knew I could never forget his sensitive, intelligent eyes and his polite, restrained demeanour.

I now realize I had developed what is known in the medical profession as transference – a mad, involuntary "Doctor-I-Worship-You-Because-You-Know-Everything-and-You-are-Helping-Me" dependence on him, but I couldn't help it. My whole life had suddenly spiralled out of control, and knowing he would come to see me every morning with hopefully better and better news always made me feel supported and inspired confidence that I would make progress. He was the consistently brightest spot of my day. And his gorgeous, wavy black mane was always a delightful distraction from my grief and guilt about not only ravaging the lives of my family, but also being completely incapable of doing anything about it.

Jean-Pierre was experiencing too much trauma himself to give me much emotional support during this stage of my recovery. In fact, he remarked that I actually bolstered him even though it was me who was in hospital. He would come see me in the evenings, exhausted and distraught from his marathon days struggling as an "I-have-No-Idea-What-the-Fuck-I'm-Doing-Mr.-Mom," while hanging onto his job as a financial analyst at Transport Canada. Most of our visits centred on handling our home and baby girl and just getting through the crisis.

* * *

That morning, when a blessed nurse freed me from the intravenous harness, I told her I would like to see Dr. Mallya before my ambulance arrived. To some extent, physiotherapy had created new pathways for my newly liberated arm to seize up in screaming agony, but my balance was now markedly improved with less support. I could now take a few steps unassisted, even though my right phantom half felt twice as heavy as the left. After the latest "encouraging" 10-minute treatment session, I was totally spent and begging for more pain meds before the every-four-hours dosing interval. Even though half of me was numb, the stinging raged relentlessly.

Lunch came and went.

Around 2 p.m., Dr. Mallya suddenly appeared. He looked harried.

"You wanted to see me?"

"Yes, I just wanted to thank you for everything."

"You're welcome," he said, and disappeared.

3

Hotel California

The ambulance driver didn't show up for me till almost 4 p.m. Friday afternoon. I was already exhausted with anxiety after waiting nearly all day.

He came in with a wheelchair and fastened the brakes near my bed.

"Do you need any help transferring?'

"I should be okay, thanks." By now, I had developed some adeptness with aiming myself toward handlebars. "Just maybe spot me while I'm standing, okay?"

"You bet," he said. "Go ahead."

I made it look as if I was an expert. At that, anyway.

"Looks like you're doing really well."

"Thanks," I said, grinning through gritted teeth. *Just focus on getting there, in one piece.* "Okay, let's do this."

When we got to the ambulance, he asked me if I would rather sit in the front seat instead of being harnessed in the rear. Surprised, I immediately said yes. The thought of being outdoors for the first time in three weeks filled me with joy, and I relished the thought of witnessing the drive through the city.

Huge mistake.

I can't even remember how he managed to hoist me up into the high cabin and fasten my seatbelt. Moving in different ways for the first time sent unbelievable shocks through parts of my body I had forgotten existed. I sucked in my breath and held it.

"Are you okay?"

I nodded insistently, even though my entire right side had seized up. I was too embarrassed to tell him that maybe I couldn't handle this and should go in the back after all, but I was also too exhausted from the horrific stinging to even consider being moved again into the back. I imagined it would probably be just as bad if not worse there, so it was better to literally grit my teeth and get through the ride as quickly as possible.

"I … just have crazy pain issues," I finally said. "Just try not to make too many sharp turns."

"Okay, I promise – no running red-lights."

"Ha ha."

The bright sunlight hurt my eyes, the buildings and houses swirled around chaotically, and I could have sworn the ambulance had no shock absorbers. Every single bump in the road brought cringe after cringe. My head pounded in protest.

Mercifully though, our ride did not last long. Shortly after turning off Bronson Avenue, we approached the dreaded Saint-Vincent Hospital, an ancient, grey stone building, four stories high, with small, thin, sparsely spaced windows. It looked like a cross between a convent and a prison.

We circled around to the back of the building and stopped in front of the admissions dock. Right next to the entrance sat a deliriously happy, wild-eyed little man in a wheelchair, wearing a bright red sweatshirt; his legs shrivelled; his head lolling back and forth while he howled with erratic joy to whatever music was playing in his head; with his huge mouth contorting in a crooked toothy, drooling grin. He didn't mean to make me feel nauseated.

J-Jesus … this must be Ottawa's version of the Eagles' Hotel California … where Don Henley's screaming … you can check out any time you want … but you can never leave …

I was freaking out inside.

The ambulance driver got me back into the wheelchair and brought me down a short hall which opened up to a large, modern, spotless reception area. We turned right and continued about half a block, past closed doors that looked like offices, and then turned right again. We had arrived. The long, dark gaping hallway about to consume me was the Stroke Rehabilitation Ward.

He wheeled me to a more brightly lit, busy nurses' station. Everyone's faces lit up with smiles as soon as they saw me, and a blond, short-haired woman with a stern, lined face that spoke of many years of hard responsibility and no nonsense immediately approached me.

"Hi, you must be Cathy," she said cheerfully. "I'm Head Nurse

Sandi Millar. How are you doing?"

"Pretty tired," I mumbled.

"I can imagine," she said, checking her watch. "It's already been a pretty long day for you." Her nod of thanks dismissed the ambulance driver, and as she took over the wheelchair, I raised my left hand in thanks as I heard him wish me good luck.

"Let's get you settled in your room and let you rest a bit, and then a couple of nurses will come see you and start our intake procedures."

Sandi wheeled me into a tiny room directly across the hall from the nursing station. A sour, frumpy old woman sat on the edge of the first single bed, staring at us with an accusatory face. She looked desperately unhappy.

"Cathy, this is your roommate Edna. Edna, this is Cathy."

"Hi, Edna."

Her cold glare unwavering, she looked like she was about to say something. "H … HELL-O," she finally said.

Sandi smiled at her, then at me. "Cathy, Edna has some trouble with her speech sometimes." Edna closed her eyes and nodded grimly. "Edna, I'm just going to close the privacy curtain between you two now. Cathy's very tired and needs to rest for a while."

She brought me over to the other tiny bed, drew the curtain shut, and got me settled on the bed.

"There we go. Pillows okay?"

"Yes. Thanks so much."

She smiled. "The intake nurses will be here fairly soon, and then your physiatrist, Dr. Clifford, will check in on you, so I'll let you rest for now."

"Fizz-I-a-trist?"

"Yes. Dr. Clifford is a physical medicine and rehabilitation specialist, known as a physiatrist, and he heads up our unit. He's a very nice man."

"Oh, okay." I had never heard of that type of doctor.

"I should also mention that supper is at 5:30. You may have noticed the two small tables and chairs just around the corner from each room. All meals are eaten at those tables in the hall. That way we can be right there to help you use your utensils if you need it, things like that."

I don't like that idea!

"Okay then, I'll leave you to rest now, but if you need anything or if anything's bothering you, here's the call button, and don't hesitate to talk to me directly at any time," she assured me. "See you later."

I closed my eyes and just tried to relax, tried not to cry. I was dealing with too many new things and too much stimulation, and I was exhausted and hurting everywhere. It even hurt to breathe. I just wanted to roll up in a ball and check out. *But this is Hotel California ... will they ever let me leave?*

Before the check-in nurses arrived, I looked around and surveyed my new surroundings. A pleasant enough south-facing window was right next to my bed, and barely more than a wheelchair width away from the end of the bed sat a shared sink with faucets. Next to it a thick, heavily glazed wooden door with a crucifix overtop opened to a raised toilet, equipped with grab bars on each side. Beside it was another identical door that Sandi had opened to put my bag inside … *so yes, that was the closet. Hmmm … it's old and small … but very clean … meticulously maintained … looks like it'll be easy enough for me to manage.*

"Hi, Cathy!"

The shrill voice interrupted my stupor. Two nurses bustled past the privacy curtain, pulled up small chairs and noisily placed themselves on each side of my bed. *Two bespectacled faces wearing cat's-eye glasses … scoping me out, as if they're about to pounce …*

"It's been a long day for you, hasn't it? How are you feeling?"

"Awful. I really need some pain meds."

"Yes, they're coming right away. What's hurting?"

"Everything," I mumbled. My head pounded. My breathing seemed too shallow. It was so hard to breathe. *Oh please, please just go away … let me sleep …*

"Okay then, we'll just double-check through everything as quickly as we can," came the soft voice.

"Your full name."

"Date of birth."

"Height? Weight? Any allergies? Previous hospital visits? None, except delivering your daughter and having tonsils out when you were 25 …"

My heart started pounding and my chest burned so hard it felt like my heart was about to jump out into my mouth. I couldn't get any air. I started gasping.

I'm having a heart attack!

"Ohmygod!" I cried. "Can't breathe! I'm dying!"

Pandemonium ensued. "GET DR. CLIFFORD! STAT!"

I heard chairs scraping. Running. Terse orders. A blood pressure monitor slapped onto me. Things were kind of a blur; I think they attached me to a portable ECG machine, and after a short time, Dr. Clifford strode in and quietly took the reins from his late-Friday-afternoon shell-shocked nursing staff. The relief amongst all of us was almost instant.

"Hi Cathy," he said kindly. "I'm Dr. Clifford. I'm sorry that our first meeting is not under better circumstances than this."

"Yeah me too," I choked.

Sporting short dark hair and aviator wire frames, he was thin and exceptionally tall – maybe six foot five. His serious expression conveyed intelligence, concern and an aura of calmness.

He lifted his stethoscope towards my chest. "I'm going to listen to your heart for a while and then check out a few other things."

We did not speak while he listened here, and there, and back again. Then he studied the report. He exuded diligence.

"Well, I have good news," he said softly. "You have not had a heart attack. It was an anxiety attack."

I didn't understand. "Anxiety?"

He nodded and pulled up a chair. "Yes. Completely understandable." His expression was reassuring. "You've been having a really rough time lately. You've had a significant stroke. You've just had a baby, and you've never been in hospital for anything serious before. You're exhausted, in pain, you have no idea what's going to happen, and you're worried about everything. Is that about right?"

I nodded morosely. He was spot on.

"Okay, here's what I think we should do. I'm going to give you an injection for your pain right now. And if you agree, I'd like to temporarily put you on a very mild tranquilizer. I think it'll make it easier for you to focus better on your physiotherapy, which will be starting Monday. Does that sound reasonable to you?"

"Yes." I felt like I needed all the help I could get.

"Good." With a reassuring smile, he proceeded to get the blessed needle ready.

"Now, it's pretty quiet here on weekends because there are no therapy sessions, and most of the patients are allowed to go home to be with their families and practise living at home again. Of course it's too soon for you to go home yet, but I think this quiet time will be a good opportunity for you to get used to your new surroundings. And I will stop by on the weekend to see how you're doing. Does that sound okay?"

"That's very kind of you." I felt embarrassed to appear so needy.

"Okay, good." I expected that would be his cue to get up and leave, but he sat back in the chair and leaned forward. "So starting Monday, you're going to have a whole team of professionals dedicated to helping you. Not just physiotherapy – you will have treatments for the pain; you'll have an occupational therapist, who will help you figure out how to do things differently; you will have your own psychologist, who you can talk with in confidence about anything; and you'll also have a social worker to help you and your family navigate through all the changes. And of course you can talk to me any time about anything."

The enormous weight on my chest lifted. This was not "Hotel

California," after all.

"So I will be going home eventually, then."

He nodded emphatically. "Oh yes, of course. You're a lot younger than anyone else here too, so I think you'll make progress quite quickly. You'll probably be here for about six to eight weeks."

"Six to eight weeks," I repeated, understanding his perspective on the meaning of "quick" progress.

"Yes, I think so. Every week, your team and I will meet to discuss how you're doing and figure out any adjustments we might need to make to better tailor your therapies. We'll also get together with you and your husband on a regular basis to give you updates and answer any questions you might have."

"Wow. That sounds great."

"Yes, we really have a great team on the ward here, and you'll get all the time you need to sort things out," he said quietly. The needle he gave me had started to take effect. I was becoming comfortably numb.

"Thanks so much, Dr. Clifford. I feel a lot better now."

"Good." He stood up. "Gaetan and Francine are the two nursing assistants on evening duty this weekend. They're very kind, and they'll be in to say hi shortly."

"Okay, thanks."

So, until Sunday," he said, as if we were old friends, and with a casual two-finger salute, he left to start his own (albeit-already-interrupted-by-me) weekend at home with his family.

For the first time, I let myself hope that there might be a way to muddle through the quagmire of my despair.

⋆ ⋆ ⋆

When I woke up, it was dark outside. The privacy curtain was pulled open, and the bed beside me was empty.

Edna must be with her family now, till Sunday night. Good for her.

The nursing assistants, Gaetan and Francine, were a delight. Both small, slight and chipper, they looked young enough to have barely finished high school. They always seemed to have a smile on their faces, were so easy to get along with, and delighted in saying things to make me chuckle.

I had missed the 5:30 p.m. dinner call due to my medically induced "nap," and like most other nights, I had trouble falling back to sleep.

"Would you like to watch a movie?" Gaetan asked me. "I could set you up in the TV room; then I'll go find you something to eat."

He helped me into a wheelchair and brought me to a large, sparse room with an old TV positioned high up near the ceiling. I had no idea what movie I was watching, but I felt giddy just to be doing something outside of my hospital cubicle.

Not much time passed before Gaetan reappeared, pushing a wheeled tray towards me. "Hope this'll tide you over till tomorrow," he said, positioning the tray over the wheelchair. On it was a small tuna sandwich on delicious crusty whole grain bread, a banana and a cup of tea.

"Wow, Gaetan – thank you so much!"

"That's another great secret about this place," he whispered, with a devilish grin. "All the food's prepared here on site – not like most other hospitals that just have their meals shipped in. This place is run by the Bruyère Sisters, and they strongly believe in serving patients the most wholesome food possible."

"Aah. So that's why there's little crucifixes all over the place."

"Yeah. And get this – every once in a while, they serve French fries made on the spot from fresh potatoes." He grinned and rubbed his hands together conspiratorially. "Sometimes they're even still sizzling when they arrive – but you may not be here long enough to get a chance to try them!"

4

Becoming Left-Handed and Left-Footed

On Saturday morning, as I was finishing my first breakfast in the hallway, the attending nurse suggested that it would be an excellent time for me to continue the transition to dressing myself independently. She shadowed me closely as I prepared to stand up, and slowly limp across the room with the pace of a snail to the end of my bedside. I plopped down.

"Phew!"

The nurse still stood next to me. She looked calm.

"Okay, I'm going to get up now and open the closet." She nodded, and waited.

I stood, then carefully moved around the corner of my bed to stand at the end of it, facing the closet. I took a deep breath, reached across, and opened the door. My lonely garment bag lay at the bottom. My right side wouldn't stop screaming at me, but I was determined. *You WILL do this.*

Favouring my left side, I leaned towards the bag and gripped it with my good hand. *Aha! Got it!* Slowly I straightened, waited to let myself breathe a few moments, then turned clockwise and took the few agonizing steps I needed to make it back safely to the bed, and successfully plopped down, bag beside me.

"Okay," I said, exhaling deeply. *Made it.* I should have been ecstatic over this small achievement, but all I felt was exhaustion.

Oh the burning the burning, this goddamn never-ending burning …

The nurse peeked around from the privacy curtain. I hadn't noticed she'd already closed it. "Okay good, Cathy. Just use the call button if you need anything."

Jean-Pierre had been instructed to bring in a couple of jogging suits for my daily rehab activities, so he had to go out and buy them for me, since I had never jogged. In 1984, jogging suits were neither as fashionable nor widely available as they are now, but bless his heart, he managed to track down some butt-ugly ones at Zellers. One was a sickly yellow; the other a pallid light blue. I pulled out the top and matching pants of the blue one, along with a bra and panties.

With a sigh, I picked up the bra. Piece of cake (sort of). Since my arms were short, I grew up fastening the back clasps in front, then turning the bra around to reposition the cups, so when I was first shown this method at the General Hospital, it was already old hat. Except now, I just had to place the correct side of the clasp into the burning numb right fingers with my left hand, and try as best

I could to hang on tight, never taking my eyes off the right hand, while my left wrestled behind my back to retrieve the other end. Quite often, the right hand couldn't hang on long enough, and the bra would flop down to the floor or onto my lap. So, I'd just try again. And again …

There! Success on the third attempt. (Sigh of relief). That wasn't too bad …

Now for the sweatshirt. Position it on my lap so that my left hand can help guide the right hand to its sleeve hole first. I can't tell where my hand is, but I see the big bump near the shoulder seam, so with my left hand, I help push the right arm carefully through its sleeve, far enough to allow my left hand to push through its armhole and then pop my head through the collar hole.

This constant do-by-sight concentration was exhausting though, just having to think about how I would make every move before doing it. *I'm never sure it will even work until I try it. Nothing comes naturally anymore. Every move that once seemed instinctive now has to be planned and thought through a different way, all the time. Makes me feel like I'm forcing myself, all the time. It makes my head hurt. And I never get a break from feeling as if half my body hates me …*

I want to lie down again, but it's only first thing in the morning, and I haven't even finished dressing my lower half yet, so I must continue …

Virtually overnight, at age 27, I felt like 87.

* * *

True to his word, Dr. Clifford showed up Sunday afternoon in jeans and a puffy greyish-green winter vest while I was trying to do a large-blocked crossword puzzle with my left hand. My sweet Jean-Pierre had brought me the book.

"Wow," Clifford said, his eyes wide. He looked impressed. "How's that going?"

"Pretty good, actually. I played classical piano and also used to play a lot of rock by ear, so my left hand's already quite agile. I've always been pretty ambidextrous, so it shouldn't be too hard for me to get used to being left-handed."

"That's great." He sat down. "Would you like our speech pathologist to bring you some writing exercise sheets?"

"Sure!"

"How do you feel on the Xanax?"

"Much better," I confirmed. "I can actually think straight now. I'm so looking forward to starting my rehab tomorrow."

"Looks to me like you've already started," he said. "Now, I just want to give you a heads- up on how things will go tomorrow. It will be a very busy day. Right after breakfast at 9, a porter will come with a wheelchair and bring you to the end of this hall, where the physiotherapy room is. Kathryne Eyre will be your physiotherapist from 9 to 10. After that, she'll escort you to the treatment centre on the left managed by Madame Paquette." He smiled. "Everyone calls her Madame Paquette. She's going to try icing your right neck, shoulder and arm to see if that calms down the stinging."

"Ice?"

"Yes. We'll see if that helps, and if it doesn't, we'll try something else. After your treatment, you'll go back to your room, have some quiet time, then lunch, and then I think around 1:30 p.m., you'll be seeing your occupational therapist. Her name is Sandra Hobson."

"Wow, you weren't kidding! I will be busy."

"Yes, your days here will go by pretty quickly during the week. Is there anything you want to ask me?"

"No, I'm good. Thanks so much for stopping by."

"My pleasure. Edna should return before 8 p.m.; that's when the weekend home visitors are supposed to be back in their rooms."

I grinned. "So, we have a curfew?"

"Ya, right," he joked. "Seriously though, I expect you'll probably be ready for your first weekend trip home in the next couple of weeks."

"Wow! Really?"

"Yes, I think so. We'll likely have a team meeting this Friday to discuss it with you and Jean-Pierre." He got up from the chair.

"I promise I'll work hard," I declared.

"Oh, I know you will," he said. "See you tomorrow."

With an easy half-smile, he did his two-fingered salute, and loped out. I still couldn't get over how friggin' tall he was!

* * *

Later that evening, around 7:30 p.m., my roommate Edna returned by herself. She appeared to be fairly mobile as she removed her winter coat and scarf and hung them up, albeit with difficulty. Short and rotund, with short, tight grey curls, her sadness remained unchanged. I made sure I was smiling when she turned and looked my way.

"Hi, Edna."

She nodded jerkily, tried to smile, but said nothing. Then she turned, moved with deliberation towards her bed, plopped down, and turned my way.

"Did you have a good weekend?" I asked.

She nodded hesitantly, and after a long pause, said, "S-so … tired."

I nodded. "I can relate to that."

"W … w … what's – y-your … BALL! … NO!! … your NAME?"

"It's Cathy." Edna's eyes lit up a little. "You get around pretty well, eh?"

She nodded, but pointed to her mouth with frustration. "It's just … THIS. I have SO much … t-trouble … trouble f-f-finding … the … the right WORDS."

"That must be so hard," I said.

She closed her eyes and sighed, nodding emphatically. "So mixed up," she murmured, and we lapsed into quiet stupor for a while, resting our wounds.

All of a sudden Edna shouted "SKYLIGHT!" – jolting me awake.

Edna, distressed, was shaking her head and rapidly waving her hand in front of her face. I had no idea what she was trying to tell me.

"Skylight?"

"NO! I mean … SKYLIGHT!" She raised her arm over her head and pointed towards the ceiling a few times. "Wh-what did … Skylight s-say?" Then she pointed at me urgently.

"Oh!" I couldn't suppress a smile. "You mean Dr. Clifford?"

"YES!" Relief washed over her, and she smiled and relaxed. We both giggled.

"Oh yeah, he's REALLY tall!"

I've always wondered if Dr. Clifford ever knew she called him that.

"I'm okay," I assured her. "I had an anxiety attack. I was so exhausted and worried about everything that I just lost it. I have a three-month old baby girl and a super stressed-out husband at home. My entire right side is numb and so heavy, and it never stops stinging."

"Oh dear," she said. "I h-have an … irregular … h-heart … and have h-had … l-lots of … lots of little … w-ones …"

"Little strokes?"

She nodded sadly and closed her eyes, and then we both settled back into our own stupors. Poor Edna.

That's when I understood why Dr. Mallya had told me that I was lucky my right-sided stroke had not left me with any communication difficulties. Aphasia is probably one of the most frustrating and demoralizing disabilities to live with. It's one of the things *Die Hard* movie star Bruce Willis struggled with before his dementia diagnosis was first made public. You may be able to walk to the washroom and use it by yourself, but if there's no more toilet paper and you can't ask for another roll, more often than not, you're kind of up "Schitt's" Creek (as in the CBC comedy series).

I experienced the devastating effects of aphasia myself after my second right-sided stroke six years later. I will never forget the expression of pure horror on Jean-Pierre's face when he first desperately tried to get me out of bed to walk, and I started babbling gibberish. I shared his horror in realizing I wasn't making any sense, but even more terrifying was that I couldn't even figure out what I was trying to tell him.

I was extremely lucky that my own speech problems after my later stroke straightened themselves out only a week later.

* * *

Monday morning, after meds, blood pressure and other checks (like did you have your BM today?) and getting dressed, I tried to ignore my constant headache and, under hawk-eyed supervision, I limped into the hallway to my designated table, clumsily sat, and focussed on getting through my first breakfast amongst the seniors on Ward 1D. None of us showed much cheer, as we were all bogged down with our own unique personal struggles while trying to relearn how to feed ourselves.

After collapsing onto the bed to recover from breakfast for too-short-a-time, a small man with a black, French-cut mop of hair and Fu Manchu mustache knocked on the doorframe and nodded at me, pushing a wheelchair my way. Wordlessly, he escorted me left to the end of the hall, past a few other sad old faces still lingering at their small dining tables, staring at what was left of their break-fasts, as if they weren't sure whether, what or how to finish.

I was raring to go, however. I had a goal. *Work hard to get well enough to be able to go home in a few weeks. And practise just to be with your baby. Just to hold her again …*

When we got to the end of the hall, a large, fully windowed room blossomed open in the sunshine. Patients lay on the floor on large mats while therapists worked on their weakened limbs; another determined man was walking herky-jerky between two support bars, his hands gripping each side with determination, as he willed himself not to look at his feet; and a prim and proper elderly lady pedalled half-heartedly on a stationary bike, looking as if she had already given up her battle.

A spritely young Asian woman with short, sassy hair smiled and approached as soon as she noticed me. "Hi. You must be Cathy," she said. "My name's Kathy too – Kathy Eyre. I'll be your physiotherapist. Let's bring you over here and get you started."

She wheeled me over to a raised mat located close to a wall, locked the chair, and asked me to transfer from the chair to the mat and sit down. By this time, I was becoming more used to people studying every move I made and telling me the safest new ways to do everything. I gathered up all these acquired tactics and training, and with shaky legs (and Kathy hovering), I stood, slowly turned 180 degrees using my left foot to lead the rotation, bent over slightly and then held on to both arms of the wheelchair, and jerkily eased myself down to a sitting position on the elevated mat. Eureka! Even through the raging burning, I did it exactly how I was supposed to.

"Excellent!" Kathy had a beautiful smile. "Let's do an assessment now to see where you're at." Again, out came the geometric measuring equipment. She had me lie down and compared my self-initiated left leg and knee movements and range of motion to those of my affected right leg, and then stretched them herself to determine how much of a difference there was. Then she did the same thing with my arms.

"Your range of motion is actually very good and you're strong," she said. "The biggest thing for you will be to get used to how differently your right side feels compared to your left."

"Yeah, you got that right."

"Now how about trying to do a bridge?" A bridge was where I laid on my back with knees bent and then lifted up my buttocks as high as I could.

"Okay boss," I said, grinning.

"Try moving your feet as far back as you can toward your bum, that's it … and now lift your bottom up just a bit … that's good … don't go for broke though … and now slowly back down. Good! … And again … ?"

* * *

After many bridges and a few other seated stretches, Kathy announced she was going to try me on a TENS machine.

"What's that?"

"TENS stands for transcutaneous electrical nerve stimulation," she explained. "It's a small device that sends very low-voltage electrical impulses through electrodes that I'll attach to your skin. Sometimes it can stimulate the nerves to provide better response, and it often can provide some pain relief." (Today, Dr. Ho's "revolutionary" electronic pain reduction devices advertised on TV are like TENS machines.)

"Heck, bring it on!"

The black, battery-powered unit was about the size of a cigarette package, with an intensity dial ranging from levels 1 to 10 and several long wires with electrodes. Kathy attached them to my neck, shoulder and upper arm with circular pink sticky tapes.

With the electrodes attached, she turned the unit on, and showed me how to regulate the dial. The TENS waves felt wonderful.

"Everyone reacts differently, so we'll start very low at first, at level 2, and once you're used to that, we'll try increasing it and see how you feel."

At first, I enjoyed the faintest ebb and flow of warm tingles. I smiled and nodded, and Kathy slowly turned it up to 3. Much stronger, warmer pulses coursed through me.

"Wow. That's crazy."

"Are you okay?"

"Yes. Crazy nice."

So she left it like that for a couple of minutes. "Want to see how it feels when it's a little stronger?"

"Sure."

She cranked it up to the fourth level.

"Ow ow – now that stings!" I was still grinning, though.

She turned it back down to 2. "We might be able to increase it as you get used to it. I'll leave you here for a few minutes and then I'll bring you to the treatment room. And tomorrow, we'll start walking."

I lay back, closed my eyes and focussed on following the pleasant, warm electric waves pulsing down the veins of my neck, shoulder and arm, trying to will away the burning and restore my sense of touch.

The relief was only temporary, though. Almost as soon as the pulses stopped, the crushing burning reared its ugly head again. I felt like there was a monster living inside me.

* * *

Pain treatment maven Madame Paquette's smile was as strong as she was. Wearing a mustard-coloured dress covered with a white chef's apron, her hefty upper arms strained the fabric of her short sleeves as she expertly wrapped my entire arm from shoulder to wrist in white towels. She had me sit next to a huge basin brimming with small ice cubes, gently positioned my arm on top, and then completely packed the ice around it.

"There," she announced, grabbing an old, yellowed egg timer and clicking the dial to the 10-minute mark. "Any more than that and you'll turn into Popsicle Pete!"

I chuckled.

"In the meantime, give me a shout if it starts to hurt or if you feel uncomfortable, okay?"

"Sure thing. Thanks."

After about a minute, the stinging became more intense, and at five minutes, a disturbing numbness set in; my arm felt leaden. It distressed me.

"Okay, Madame Paquette," I chirped, after about six minutes, "I think it's time to free Popsicle Pete."

"No worries," she said, and dug out the arm. "Sometimes it can take a few treatments to get used to it. Want to try again tomorrow?"

"Sure," I said, but she could see I was discouraged. I knew almost instantly that ice was not going to help. My diagnosis later confirmed that in combination with astereognosis (the inability to know what you're touching without looking at it), I was also unusually hypersensitive to hot and cold. My thalamus, the part of the brain that controls the five senses, had been turned so haywire that I wondered if I could ever get used to my new self. To this day, when I'm near a hot stove, my right side will feel the oven's heat before the left does, and even the slightest cool breeze will send waves of painful electric shocks through my neck and down my arm.

Only recently, in 2021, after reading *Sentient,* by genius BBC zoologist Jackie Higgins, I was amazed to discover that people who lack awareness of the location of their body parts, and experience only heat, cold and pain are now diagnosed as lacking proprioception, which is now scientifically considered to be a "sixth" sense. When you're never sure where your body parts are, you have to keep checking yourself visually, and this can affect your posture, balance and fine motor skills.

For example, whenever I drive these days, I always wear a water backpack, because I can grab the hose to suck on the mouthpiece with my right hand while my left hand continues to control the steering wheel, instead of numbly trying to grasp for a bottle and risk taking my eyes off the road.

"Heat may also work better," Madame Paquette added. "We can try you in the hot tub."

A porter brought me back to my room, and I crashed on my bed, exhausted, until we were summoned back into the hallway for another stab-and-grab lunch.

Shortly after lunch, a speech pathologist dropped by to give me some writing practice exercise sheets.

"Dr. Clifford told me you're already doing quite well adjusting to writing with your left hand," she said. There was never any discussion about torturing my right hand to try to get it to write. It still came naturally for me to clumsily grip a knife with my right hand to cut food because I could primarily use my wrist to manipulate the knife, rather than the fingers, which could only maintain limited grasping, being dead-to-the-touch. The knife usually fell to the floor a few times during every meal, but it was good for me to bend down at the waist while seated and reach across to pick it up with my left (and of course wipe it with my napkin).

I nodded. "I've always been kind of ambidextrous from piano playing."

"That's wonderful," she said. "I've brought you a bunch of exercises you can work with that may help with letter formations and connections. Keeping a diary is a good way to practise too."

"Oh, that's a great idea. Thank you," I said. So I began to keep a journal. I have no idea what happened to it, though.

She passed me her business card, but I later lost it, and thus, I can't remember her name today. "Don't hesitate to contact me if you have any questions, but I'm sure you'll do just fine."

* * *

The wheelchair trip to occupational therapy was a long one, to a different part of the hospital. Another expansive room greeted me with sunny windows, a mini-kitchen area with a sink, counter and cupboards, several tables topped with all sorts of art and woodworking projects, and other strange equipment I had never seen before.

Sandra Hobson looked up from a heavy-duty sewing machine,

smiled, and came over. Serious and kind, she always wore a white medical coat, her brown hair always piled high.

The porter silently left, and Sandra wheeled me to a more appropriate spot for us to chat.

"I hear you've got a beautiful little baby girl at home," she said. I nodded sadly. She asked me her name, I told her, and she smiled.

"That's beautiful. I've been thinking about ways we can help you get back to caring for her independently." My eyes lit up.

"What would you think if I made you a sandbag of her approximate size and weight, perhaps a little heavier? Then, you could practise different ways to carry her, perhaps against your left hip, or something like that."

"Wow! That's a great idea!" My heart surged with hope. I could do this. I WOULD do this. (After relearning how to walk, of course).

Sandra scribbled down a few notes. "Okay, then. We'll have a lot of fun with that."

She got up, still serious, and came back with a large, paper lunch bag.

Oh, no. Not again …

"Now I know you've had this test done before at the General Hospital to assess the sensation loss in your hand, but I'm going to make a similar assessment as to how it affects your dexterity. And since some time has passed, you never know; it may have changed a bit."

I nodded. I needed to know myself and learn my limitations.

Unfortunately, nothing had changed. If anything, my angry, injured brain seemed to be making my numb hand sting even more violently whenever it touched something in the bag, and I still had absolutely no clue what I was touching or trying to grasp, let alone discern which fingers were moving. Maybe it was the morning ice treatment. Maybe it was the extreme fatigue from my busy morning. I had no idea. At this point, nobody else did, either. My previous joy from learning about my soon-to-be-gestating sandbag baby slowly evaporated with every failed attempt at trying to grasp "the little ball" or "the keychain."

Sandra scribbled some more notes. All business.

"I understand you've started writing with your left hand. How's that going?"

"Surprisingly well. The speech pathologist just dropped off some exercises for me, and I'm going to start keeping a diary."

"Oh, very good," she said. "Do as much as you can, whenever you can."

"I will."

"Excellent. You're looking tired."

I nodded.

"I just want to quickly go over one last thing with you before I call the porter to take you back to your room. Something else we've been doing here lately is making a kind of "sling" for our stroke patients."

"A sling?"

"Yes, I'll show you one I'm almost finished making." She turned around and retrieved a strange multi-strapped fabric and Velcro contraption from the table behind her. "This white foam cylinder here fits under your right armpit. It helps maintain space between your arm and shoulder, and can prevent pain caused by muscle shrinkage from lack of use, which can lead to things like "frozen shoulder." The sling supports your arm, makes it feel lighter and takes weight off the shoulder too."

"Oh, that'll be nice. Will I be wearing it all the time?"

"Well not to bed and probably not for physio, and we'll see how you tolerate it. I'll definitely have it ready for you this week, so you'll have some time to experiment and see how you feel with it before you start going home on weekends."

Wow. I would be going home on weekends soon! I couldn't wait; yet, while much calmer on the Xanax, I was still terrified.

"Once you're a bit stronger, and you've been home a few weekends, you and I can go to your place for half a day during the week, when there'll be no distractions, and you can prepare something in the kitchen."

"Let's make baby food! I have a food processor."

"Sure! We can also make you special tools for the kitchen too, if you need them – like a cutting board with a ridge on the side, or we can add a nail sticking upwards to anchor fruits or veggies to make it easier to cut."

⋆ ⋆ ⋆

When I was brought back into my room, I gasped.

Someone had done a makeover of my room. Beautiful photos of my darling baby were tacked on the wall around my bed. Oh, how I drank in her eyes, her sweet face, her tiny hands, her little clenched fists … and there were so many cards, letters and a few floral arrangements on the windowsill. Gosh, so many people were rooting for me!

As soon as the porter left, I burst into tears. It was just too much for me to bear all at once. Exhausted with conflicting emotions of elation, love, guilt, hope and despair, I knew they were trying to help me believe in myself, to understand that I could and would become a renewed mother again. A REALLY DIFFERENT renewed mother. But how could I be a good Mom when I hadn't even learned how to walk by myself yet?

I lay down and buzzed for some more pain meds.

"In another 20 minutes," Sandi Millar told me. I closed my eyes, curled up like a fetus and waited. I knew I had no choice but to wait for everyone else to take care of me now. I had no idea I was developing the patience I needed in order to make long-term progress. It rankled me, being so dependent on others, and not knowing how things were going to turn out. But I had no choice; I had to rely on others in order to become independent again.

Later, after a drug-lulled rest, I got up and went over to the windowsill for some encouragement. The largest, most ornate bouquet came from my employer, the Communications Branch of EDC. "Get Well Soon," was all the tag said.

Hmmm, how eloquent …

With the bouquet, I found a card from my colleagues with a similarly banal printed message and about 25 signatures. No personal words of encouragement, not even from my manager. Ominous. They obviously had no idea what they were going to do with me. Heck, I had no idea what I was going to do with me.

In 1984, six months was all the time off provided for maternity leave, and I was well into the fourth month by now, so I knew I would have to go on some form of disability leave, but that was the least of my worries. Right then, I couldn't even imagine how I would work again.

This challenge got me thinking about all the challenges I had faced and overcome in my determination to do everything I could to become a professional communicator.

I dropped out of the journalism program at Carleton University before Christmas in first year because of "The Pill." The oral contraceptive prescribed to me caused severe hemorrhaging. It made me so anemic and I missed so much time, I couldn't handle my studies along with the total two-hour daily bus commute. I had chosen to live in a rooming house with a couple of batty old ladies for $70 per month, since it was close to my high school sweetheart and financed by my parents, who had moved back to Coquitlam, B.C., the previous year. To make a long story short, my uber conservative parents were so absorbed with their own struggles that they never gave my older brother Fred and me much useful advice or support.

From a very young age, I can remember my Dad would grin like Jack Nicholson and curse, "Children are supposed to be seen and not heard," as if he was joking. But he wasn't. He'd also quip, "I know everything," because he really thought he did. But he didn't. Even in the 1990s, he once told me in earnest that he hated hiring women because "they just went off and got pregnant."

My parents hardly talked to each other, but they both yelled at us a lot. I sucked my thumb till I was five years old. I was always being told to "pipe down." My poor dear Mom, forced to abandon her dreams of becoming a ballerina after a heart defect discovered in her teens, became a school teacher. She quit work when she became a mother and returned to substitute teaching when my brother and I were both in high school. She enforced family rules using guilt tactics.

In my early teens, she'd shift her long, sad, victimized stare my way and nag me to lose weight and "hold my tummy in" (as she had learned in ballet) to look more appealing; yet every time she knew I was leaving the house to meet up with a boy or go on a date, her fearful, repetitive whining "don't have intercourse until you're married" warnings simultaneously enraged and inhibited me.

Fred and I loved grooving to rock LPs on Dad's awesome Sony stereo after school on days when both parents were at work, but as soon as we heard the Ford Custom growling up the gravel driveway, we bolted to shut off the music before the front door opened, especially if it was Led Zeppelin's *Whole Lotta Love* or *The Lemon Song*. Otherwise, he would storm in and bellow "TURN OFF THAT GALL-DARNED GARBAGE RIGHT NOW!!

Then all of a sudden, my father quit his job and announced to us that they were moving back to Vancouver. Fred and I couldn't wait to escape our stressful environment, and we gleefully took the opportunity to stay in Ottawa and live our own lives, free of our parents' leaden pressures.

After dropping out of Carleton, I took the first decent-paying steno job I could find to support myself, becoming a secretary at the Anti-Inflation Board, for the Director of the Data

Management Division.

I felt I had let myself down.

A secretary was the last thing I wanted to be; to me it was such a sexually stereotypical occupation, but given my limited qualifications, I didn't have much choice. The starting salary, in 1976, was $7,808.

After a couple of years there, I scored a transfer to a more interesting assignment, working for Carole Peacock, Chief of Media Relations at Health and Welfare Canada. It was a fast-paced, dynamic environment where I helped issue news releases, and I learned a great deal. My dream was to get into advertising, and Assistant Director Lyle Cameron told me I'd probably have to move to Toronto if I wanted to get into advertising without a degree. I didn't want to move to Toronto, so eventually I decided to enroll in Public Administration at the University of Ottawa at night school. And that's where I met my future husband.

Jean-Pierre was in my class two years in a row. The first year, we just traded a few sweet barbs. I liked him. The second year, we ended up sitting together, along with his friend Laurent Bernard. At that time I was in a relationship I never should have started with a colleague from the Anti-Inflation Board who was 10 years older than me. I had stumbled into that unhealthy relationship on the rebound from a very sad and confusing breakup with the love of my life from high school.

After losing my high school sweetheart, I remember sitting on a park bench one lunch hour, resolving that my biggest goal was to save my money so I could buy myself a house in case I never met anyone else. I was so naive. (By the late '70s, premarital sex was the norm, so I chose to keep my prying but well-meaning mother in the dark about my love life. It also helped that my parents were far away on the West Coast.)

Jean-Pierre and I lived together for a couple of years before I pushed him to pop the question because we wanted to have a family, but never had I ever considered being a stay-at-home Mom. I guess only time would tell.

* * *

In my room at Saint-Vincent's, I took in the mountain of get-well cards and was blown away. Some with personal messages came from a few close EDC colleagues, as well as some surprisingly touching messages from others outside the branch who barely knew me. Friends, family and others from the distant past surprised me with sweet messages and even rambling letters of encouragement. They gave me hope, for what, exactly, I wasn't sure, but knowing that so many took the time to let me know they cared was indeed uplifting.

That night, after supper, Jean-Pierre arrived with "ma petite bébé." She looked very alert and content, whereas JP looked heart-broken, nervous and exhausted.

"Ah, wow," he said softly, regarding the baby pictures, flowers and cards. "It looks almost festive in here."

We soon found a way for me to "hold" her. JP could put her in the crook of my left arm and then position himself snugly against my left side, creating a buffer, and it worked! It felt SO good to have them next to me, smelling her soft pink skin and watching her big eyes looking up at me, as if to say *I know you're my Mommy, but how come I don't hardly see you anymore?*

She was such a calm baby.

My memories of early motherhood before the stroke are quite vague. I spent so much time in hospital, away from my baby girl, and I missed so much of her early rapid development that I had no choice but to suppress those desperate longings for her in order to survive. To this day, being excluded from so much of her infancy can bring me overwhelming sadness.

Even hearing JP talk about Debra, her husband Doug, and their daughters, Kyla and Kessa, made me feel desolate, fearful and envious. I had never met any of these people, yet my darling baby stayed with them in their home five days a week, while my hubby tried to concentrate on his financial analysis internment at Transport Canada.

Almost every day during his lunch hour, JP appeared for his "vent visit," as in venting about his problems at work. Saint-Vincent Hospital was just a 10-minute walk from his office in Place de Ville, at Kent and Sparks Street. He needed this time with me to lament about the difficulties he was having with his horrid new boss. Apparently, she had the people skills of a vulture. While several official grievances had already been filed against her for being combative, unfair, nit-picking and pushy, her allegedly abusive behaviour appeared to be escalating.

With his work troubles adding to his already exhaustive "Mom-Dad" worries, he needed to rant to fend off a complete meltdown. Heck, I had an army of people looking after me. So most of the time, I would clasp his hand, just listen, and try to be as supportive as I could be from my hospital bed. He needed me, and that helped give me a sense of purpose and a belief that I was contributing to the survival of our family.

Once his daily office torture was over, and JP got himself and our treasure back home after work, the gruelling, one-man domestic marathon of feeding, cleaning and caring for her overwhelmed him. He often felt like he had no idea what he was doing. During those lunchtime visits, I got used to being the more supportive one; he was all alone and needed reassurance from me that he was handling everything the way he should be. He did a marvellous job though. I still can't imagine how he coped.

Later, he told me that during this terrible time, he was driving home one night with our daughter fast asleep and safely bundled up in the back seat, and he was feeling particularly despondent. He turned on the car radio to CHEZ 106 FM, and a song called *Send Me an Angel* by Real Life began playing. He felt that they were singing directly to him.

Send me an angel … send me an angel … right now … right now …

He started to cry. But it was during those moments that he realized he had already been sent an angel, and the remaining tears he shed were tears of joy. Our dear, sweet baby girl was his guardian angel. He felt so blessed that she was in our lives now, and he would do everything he could to love, protect and nurture her, no matter what.

They were both my angels, too. My reasons to never give up.

* * *

Psychologist Céline Paris, another cherished member of my treatment team, quickly became a trusted confidante. I spent many hours with her, often in tears, raging about missing out on sacred mothering time, the inability to feel what I touch, my fears I would never play piano again, the never-ending burning and the overwhelming fatigue – combined with frightening dread about not being able to climb stairs, cook a meal or care for my daughter like a "normal" mom as she grew up and the goring guilt over abandoning the two most important people in my life. How long was it going to take for me to get back home? How would I be able to shop for groceries? How would I even be able to take care of myself? A mountain of anger about my own fractured relationship with my mother also erupted in nuclear fashion during those sessions.

Céline made me feel like she understood everything, and in her relaxed, professional manner, she was a truly beautiful, caring person. Simple, yet vivacious, she was down-to-earth and had a terrific sense of humour. She laughed heartily at even my silliest jokes about feeling like a senior citizen at 27; yet, she was insightful, calming and practical, and at the same time, she encouraged me to keep on dreaming.

She even suggested I should write a book about my experiences. I replied that I didn't know if I would ever be ready to do that because I needed to focus on rebuilding my unknown future with positivity, rather than waste energy wallowing in self-pity. I never got to tell Céline how much she helped me heal emotionally. She was my lifeline for months. I could bare my soul with her in ways

I couldn't with anyone else.

After my second stroke six years later, Céline had moved on from Saint-Vincent to the Riverside Hospital, but she had left me a short handwritten message on a yellow post-it note for head nurse Sandi Millar to give to me upon my second admission to Saint-Vincent. It went like this:

Dear Cathy,

I dropped by the ward to say hi to everyone today, and was devastated to learn that you had another stroke. While I'm not here to support you, please know that I am with you in my heart, and I KNOW you will be okay. Céline xo

What were the odds of her visiting just a day before my return to Hotel California? It was like a tiny bird flitting by, dropping a seed to elevate my soul.

Back to my first stroke: Claudia Newman, my social worker, wore her brown curls in layers and looked like she could have gone to Woodstock in 1969. We spent most of our visits talking about my weekend visits home and reintegrating to "normal" life, as in going back to work. She was practical and congenial, and I liked her a lot.

★ ★ ★

Every day now, I achieved new feats: walking longer and longer distances unaided; not dropping any utensils on the floor as much during mealtime; and tying my running shoes with both hands into a full bow. I wore my "sling" most of the day, and it provided some relief for the first few weeks. In occupational therapy, I practised carrying the sandbag against my left hip, but I found it to be unnaturally heavy. My right side remained a nebulous yet angry, pulsating ton of bricks, and any extra compensation from my stronger left side to maintain my balance added to the fatigue.

After about a week of ice treatments for the chronic burning, I reported to Dr. Clifford that the cold temperatures seemed to increase my numbness and made the pain worse, and I expressed a desire to try the hot tub. He agreed, and Jean-Pierre promptly brought in a bathing suit for me.

The next morning, Madame Paquette was all smiles.

"Got your swimsuit on?"

"You bet!" I unlocked the brakes on the wheelchair, wavered to my feet, thanked the porter, and Madame Paquette guided me towards a small but deep metal cylinder full of frothy warm bub-bling water. I have no recollection of how she helped me climb up and in, but ahh … it felt wonderful. The warm water also made my affected arm feel so much lighter. Ahh, floating arms felt fantastic!

Unfortunately, this bliss lasted only a few days.

I was in the tub after physio one morning, eyes closed, revelling in relaxation. But when I opened my eyes, I gasped.

The water was rapidly turning red.

Oh shit … my period … it's back!

I had completely forgotten that after giving birth and finishing nursing, several months can pass before the menstrual cycle resumes. For me, and everyone else caring for me, the stroke rehabilitation process had again overtaken my maternal recovery. I was so embarrassed.

"Mme Paquette … , " I croaked. The second time I called her, she looked up, came over, saw the red water, and her eyes widened. She froze.

"Oh my!" She blurted out.

"I'm so sorry," I said softly, near tears. "I had no idea."

Madame Paquette morphed into Sergeant Major mode, giving me soft but stern commands, as if there was no time to lose. "Well come on then. Let's get you out. Wipe you off and wrap you up. Then we'll get you to your room to shower, find you some pads AND THEN I'VE GOT TO DISINFECT THIS TUB!!!"

She didn't mean to make me feel like a "bad dog," but I did, even though she kindly bundled me up with towels in the wheelchair and speed-wheeled me back to my room. No calling a porter for this bloody assignment!

Edna's and my bathroom included a shower stall behind the toilet with a white plasticky webbed seat and supportive back, surrounded by huge handrails. Madame Paquette brought me directly to the shower seat and supervised my transfer to it from the wheelchair.

"You get cleaned up, and I'll go get you some extra towels and some pads." She took hold of the shower curtain. "You're okay for now, then?"

I nodded in shame and whispered thanks, and like the hospital's efficient sergeant, she nodded back, and rumbled out with the soiled wheelchair.

The shower washed away all my blood, sweat and tears, but not my dejection. I hung up the wet bathing suit, carefully opened the curtain and hobbled out, to find a lovely pile of fluffy white towels and a few menstrual pads. I'll have to get JP to bring me a box, I thought, as I wrapped a towel around me and turned the corner of the bathroom to my closet.

Mercifully, Madame Paquette had closed the room-divider curtain so that I had privacy to root through the closet for my underwear, ugly yellow jogging suit and running shoes. I tossed them one by one onto the bed and sat down to get dressed. It was so exhausting, especially with the extra dampness; this was already the second time I'd had to get dressed this morning, and getting the stupid big fat fucking pad placed properly inside my panties … what a nightmare! I collapsed onto the bed with a huge sigh and curled up, exhausted, ashamed, angry and upset with myself, while the stinging on the right side of my face, neck and arm raged on and on and on, down through to my fingertips …

"Y-y-you okay?" I heard Edna ask shyly.

"Yes, thanks," I mumbled. "Just resting for a while."

"Th-th-the-that's good."

✶ ✶ ✶

Shortly before lunchtime, I heard Dr. Clifford say, "Can I come in?"

I sat up to find his head poking around the corner of the privacy curtain.

"Of course."

"I just wanted to apologize on behalf of Madame Paquette for what happened this morning," he said.

"Oh, there's no need for that," I insisted, surprised and touched by his candour. "It was amazing how she took charge and handled everything."

"Well, that's really good to hear," he said. "We don't have that much experience with postpartum patients, let alone your younger age group," he explained. "So please don't hesitate to tell me at any time if there's ever anything else that comes up that you think we need to address, okay?" He was so forthright.

"Sure, but you'll probably figure it out before me anyway," I joked.

Dr. Clifford smiled. "Well I'm glad to hear it all worked out, then. See you later. Do you want the curtain open?"

"Sure, thanks."

Edna was smiling. Right after he left, I could tell she was getting ready to say something.

"D – Sk … Doctor Skylight … he's s- so nice … "

"Yes, he sure is." I was smiling now too.

* * *

My brother, Fred Roberts, bumbled in for a quick visit just before suppertime. He was still wearing the same old, yellowed, ratty fake fur coat that Mom made for him when he was in university, and with his shaggy pure white hair, crooked wire glasses and stained teeth, he had the aura of a wild animal.

It was no wonder then that soon after Fred left, dear Edna asked, "W-w … what did the … sh-sh-sheepdog say?"

* * *

After a couple of weeks, my rehab care team informed us at the Friday meeting that they thought I might be ready for my first weekend home visit the following Friday.

I could now jerkily walk the length of Ward 1D close to the wall's guardrails without accompaniment, and do about half the hallway carrying the 12-pound sandbag baby against my hip. The sandbag was indeed good practice, but I never got truly comfortable with the against-the-hip method. I found I could go farther and safer by balancing the weight in the crook of my left arm; that gave my left leg much more freedom to keep me balanced and upright.

For the next five days, relearning how to safely use stairs became the biggest challenge for me before I could be sprung for my first wild weekend at home.

First thing Monday morning, physiotherapist Kathy brought me to a stairwell between floors in the wheelchair.

"A good thing to remember is that when you're going upstairs, you should always lead with your strong leg," she explained. "And when you go down, your weaker leg should go first." She grinned. "I know a little saying that often helps. With every step you take, say to yourself: 'good leg goes to heaven; bad leg goes to hell.'"

"Good leg goes to heaven; bad leg goes to hell," I repeated. "Yeah, that'll work." (Little did I know I'd still be using this great little mantra to this very day. Even now, I nearly always "think-talk" to my affected right side before I start to do anything.)

I grabbed the round metal handrail on the wall to the right. As always, sparks of lightning drilled up through my arm, and I sucked in a quick breath. While I was learning to anticipate these nasty spikes of pain, I was still light years away from ever getting used to it, or acquiring little tricks to manage it. While I have learned how to calm down the burning sensations considerably over the years, they remain the most tiring thing to cope with.

"What are the railings like in your home?" Kathy asked me.

I thought for a moment. "They're wood, with a smaller circumference, so they should be easier."

"Okay, great. Ready?"

I nodded.

"Okay, good leg goes to heaven." I placed my left foot on the first stair. "For now, we'll only do one stair at a time, so just bring your right leg up beside the left. That's it – good! And one more … excellent!"

It was a good call to start the process one stair at a time. The effort it took to lift the leaden right knee upwards from the hip made me feel like I was a crane operator lifting an elephant on a windy day; nebulous sparks flew all over as I vice-gripped the banister and heaved upwards. Good thing I was strong and my left side anchored me.

We did five more one-at-a-time stairs, and then Kathy told me to take a break.

"That was excellent!" Kathy said, standing away from me on the floor. "How'd it feel?"

"Pretty good, but I'm gassed."

"Let's take a little break then and start thinking about how you'll get back down." She sprinted up to my level.

"Get as close to the wall as you can. That's it. Now I'm just going to spot you while you reach over to the handrail with your left hand … good. Now keep both hands on the railing, and whenever you're ready, pivot with your left foot slowly, and release your right hand."

Ouch! Oh, hell! Reaching my left arm across my chest brought angry waves of pins and needles coursing down the right side of my body, and I had no clue where my hip or right leg were or how they were not cooperating with each other. I had to look down to check on it and felt my head spin. Kathy was right next to me though, to brace me if needed, but I got the stinging right foot down beside the left, unassisted! It hurt like hell, but oh, what a rush!!!

"Ha ha!" Kathy cheered, as I stood tall and breathed deeply, ready to attempt the descent.

"So, guess what happens now?" she asked.

I smiled. "Bad leg goes to hell, right?"

"You got it. Then bring your left leg down to the same step. Ready?"

I nodded.

"Okay. Go. Slow."

I tensed my left side, released the right leg from the stair, and started to let it drop down. Strangely, it was much more difficult to lead from the right side, because it required such deep concentration to drop my foot downwards where I wanted to put it, and because I had no sense of where it was, I dared not take my eyes off it. When it landed, yet another previously unknown variety of screaming jeebies coursed up my leg. But I could see that the foot had made safe contact, and that was good.

More new shouts of protest came from the right side as soon as it realized it needed to hold the rest of my body upright before I could take my left foot off the stair and down through mid-air before it could rest beside the other foot. I felt elated though.

Each descending stair required the same grimacing focus. But

I made it to the bottom, all by myself. I heaved a huge sigh of relief.

"Whew! That was brutal!"

"But an excellent first-time effort, Cathy. How do you feel?"

I managed a small smile, but I was so tired I could hardly stand. "Pretty weak and my head's pounding," I said in a small voice. "I think I need to lie down."

"No worries." Kathy looked pleased. I got back into the wheelchair, trying my best not to plop down with too much of a thud. She pulled open the door to the ward and brought me back to my room.

Before I made the transfer from the chair to the bed, I smiled at her. "I guess this means I can go for my first home visit this weekend."

"Yes indeed, Cathy! Congrats!"

(Almost 40 years later, my family doctor, Elie Skaff, called me a "ballerina" for insisting on climbing down unassisted from the examining table onto a footstool and swinging my compromised leg around (in sync by now) without any help. He does spot me, though, which I tolerate.)

⁎ ⁎ ⁎

Wednesday morning after breakfast, occupational therapist Sandra Hobson and I climbed into a taxi at the hospital's main entrance. We were on our way to the Allard townhouse in Blair Estates for my first kitchen exercise.

Sandra confirmed the home visit with JP and me at the therapists' team meeting the previous Friday, and I had indicated I wanted to prepare some frozen baby food for our pup.

"What do you have in mind?" Sandra asked.

"Well, she's on pablum right now, and she'll be ready to start vegetables soon … so maybe I could cook and purée something fresh for her, like green beans, and then freeze them in ice cube trays. Then in the morning, Jean-Pierre can put one in a Ziploc bag for Debra to feed her for lunch."

"That sounds like an excellent plan," said Dr. Clifford. Jean-Pierre and Sandra nodded in agreement, and Céline Paris and Claudia Newman were all smiles.

"I'll get the green beans and leave the food processor on the counter for you," JP offered. "Oh, and remind me to give you a house key, Cath."

Yes sir! All systems go!

* * *

It felt so crazy to be limping up the driveway under the supervision of a relative stranger, after being away for eight long, traumatic weeks, but I was brimming with enthusiasm. I was going to act like a real Mom again, even if only for an hour or two!

Sandra wound her right arm through my left, and we climbed the two stairs together to reach the landing. I had put the house key in the left pocket of my coat ahead of time, for easy access. I inserted the key into the lock, turned it, and opened the door.

Okay, good leg, now go to heaven.

With my right hand protesting against the doorway, I raised my left foot high and long, took a huge step over the threshold (definitely not the romantic kind), then coaxed my numb knee to bend up high enough to drag the rest of its cranky lower sister foot along with it. *There,* I thought as I caught my breath. *I'm inside.*

Sandra turned on the light to see the tiled foyer better. "Nice place."

"Yeah, except for the orange shag carpet," I joked. I turned around and slid the closet door open. *Ow ow ow.* I was on a Mama Mission *(impossible?). Ignore all screaming jeebies. First order is Figure out How to Take Your Coat Off For the First Time.*

Sandra found a couple of hangers, put her long coat away first, and then waited with the other hanger ready for me just as I had finished wriggling out of the right sleeve. I struggled to get the coat haphazardly placed on the hanger myself, and then Sandra took it from me and hung it up.

"Thanks, Sandra. Kitchen's on your first left." I let her go ahead of me and took a moment to calm my breath and reorient myself. At the opposite corner of the foyer, a flight of stairs led to the second floor, and directly in front of me, the obscenely orange shaggy hallway joined up with a combined L-shaped living-dining room. There, three huge side-by-side windows took up most of the back wall, opening to a beautiful courtyard of tall trees amid rolling snow-covered grass hills, hiding the street behind it. I took a few steps toward the entrance of the large square kitchen, and despite my grief, searing pain and multiple fears, I felt giddy to finally be back home.

But when I reached the kitchen, I sucked in a breath and froze.

The Yamaha walnut spinet piano jeered at me from the living room on my right. It just stared, wooden, unsmiling, its long black and white fangs begging me to come over, sit down, and get savagely bitten.

Today was not the day to submit my deadened, angry right hand to any musical torture, though. I knew my fingers would never again be able to flicker instinctively over the upper octaves like they used to – deftly fingering the opening bars to giant hits like *Tiny Dancer,* as if I was Elton John; my jaunty rendition of Deep Purple's *Wring that Neck,* with its pounding bass chords on the left; or the honky-tonk accompaniment to Paul McCartney crooning *"No one ever left alive in nineteen hundred and eighty-five"* … that kind of musical torture. Darn good thing I'd never played that eerie tune *1984,* by David Bowie, with its foreboding message to "beware the savage jaw of 1984" …

And turns out I was right; I was never able to play again. I sat at the keyboard many times during the first few years, but the fingers on my right hand couldn't even hit the proper keys in a single phrase, let alone coordinate with the left hand. My mind knew what to play, but the short-circuits in my brain barely allowed the choppy fingers of my formerly dominant hand to complete a bar of any piece of music before the hand seized up. I had no choice but to become resigned to this new reality.

It was a good thing there were so many other essential activities of living I had to relearn that allowed me to block out the sadness about losing this gift, most of the time. However, if I heard a song I used to bang out with glee in Grade 13, such as Elton John's *Tiny Dancer,* my mind would start to play along, and sometimes I would even mime playing it, before ceasing from the fatigue of hopelessness. After all, being sad about anything for too long was never in my DNA.

After three years, I could look at the piano as a nice piece of furniture that I had tons of fun and great passion with, and maybe one day someone else would –

Sandra casually broke the spell. "You okay?"

"Oh, sure." I finally came into the kitchen. "It's just surreal seeing the piano again … I've been playing it since I was a little girl, and I was pretty good at playing by ear. I loved playing rock at school and at parties."

Sandra nodded. "That must stir up a lot inside."

I nodded sadly, and inspected the food processor. "Anyway, this is what we're here for, so I'll dig out the green beans."

I grabbed the fridge door handle with my right hand and her-ky-jerky-yanked it open, way harder than necessary. *Oh stop it burning burning … and now more and more and more burning from the frigid air – JUST IGNORE IT … JUST TRY TO IGNORE IT!!)*

I spotted the green beans in a plastic bag near the top of the crisper, pulled them out, and put the bag on the counter. Then I just stood still for a moment. It was okay to go slow, I told myself.

I found the knot to untie the clear plastic bag, and smiled. As usual, my wonderful husband had knotted it shut so tightly that it was a fight for me to get it open even at the best of times. So as usual, I just tore the bag open.

I scowled upon discovering that most of the green beans were no longer green, but dotted with grotesque brown spots and shrunken, curly ends. JP probably did the groceries on the weekend. No fault of his. Just not a good time of year.

"Yuck," I said. "These look disgusting. I'll probably have to toss half of them, and the rest are going to need major trimming."

"Oh well, at least it'll all be great practice," Sandra said cheerfully. She took a seat at the kitchen table and settled in.

I clumsily selected my favourite paring knife from the cutlery drawer, backed up and bent over slightly to withdraw the cutting board and a colander from a lower cupboard, always trying to lead with my right side. Every movement stung in a new and different way, but as had been stressed to me from day one, I had to try to use my affected side as much as possible. This can be supremely difficult when you instinctively want to initiate every movement with your more dominant side. And avoid pain. It's just easier. Every movement exhausted me, but I just kept silently repeating *You are strong. You can do this. You must Use it or Lose it. Use it or Lose it …*

Safety always took precedence, though. I picked up the knife with my left hand, and carefully positioned it into my right palm. Fascinated, I watched my numb fingers safely curl around it and grip firmly enough for cutting . I jerkily circled the wrist a few times, grimacing and trying to figure out what kinds of pins and needles the knife triggered in response to the stimuli. Once satisfied that the knife probably wouldn't unexpectedly shift quickly enough to cut off the left fingers in my compromised grip, I picked up the first decaying bean with my left hand. Holding it steady, I chopped off both ends as smoothly as I could with my right hand, and then cut out an inedible part in the middle. The left hand quickly picked up the pieces and tossed the remaining acceptable fragments into the colander.

With a squawk, I dropped the knife onto the counter and shook out my hand. My spastic hand was on fire all the way up through the arm and felt like it was about to drop off at the shoulder.

"Oof, that was tough." I paused and considered whether I should try using the knife with my left hand … but since birth, my right hand held the knife at mealtime. Especially important now. Keeping the fork in the left hand provided a steady anchor for the food while the right hand hacked away.

I picked up the knife with my left hand. *Oh, that feels so much better!* But when I picked up the bean with my right hand and placed it on the cutting board, I stopped.

"Oh … shit … Sandra, I don't think I have enough control to hold the bean still long enough, without my hand jerking. I might cut myself!"

"You're probably right," she said softly. "At least for now. And like I said before, we can always make you a cutting board with a nail sticking upwards, so you can anchor food on it if you ever want to cut using your left hand."

I nodded, and got back to business. Bean by brownish bean, each piece became a wee bit easier to prune, and before I knew it, I had established a new, better, slower rhythm, and hey … the colander was full!

Buoyed by my success with the paring knife, I gripped the weighted plastic handle with both hands, and with arms stretched out, carefully navigated the few required steps to rest in front of the steel sink. *Holy cow, I feel like I'm auditioning for Cirque du*

Soleil! Every move involves risk assessment!

*Okay, turn on the tap. Yeah, your right hand can do this solo. Ugh … oh why don't you go fuck off, you fucking exhausting stingers … Hah! Ow! Good, the beans are rinsed; now let them drain in the sink while you retrieve a saucepan. Yeah, okay, now sidestep over to the cupboard. Hmm, in this kitchen it Hurts So Good, John Mellencamp … Yes right hand, grab the door handle, and pull. Ow! Yes, untangle that stupid middle finger. Ow ow ow! Okay, there's the pot. Bend both knees, just a bit, together now, ow ow, now reach gently … ow ow … okay. Now the robot walk; back to the sink, yes, and you gotta keep on holding on tight to that pot. Squeeze it in beside the colander. Yowszers! F***off, stings! Reset. Rest. Breathe. Good. Right hand on to the pot; flip the beans into it from your left. Ow! Toss the colander on the counter. Ow. Good. Ow … at least it Hurts So Good!*

After about five minutes, with the beans lovingly blanched and cooled in the colander under a stream of cold water, I located an empty ice cube tray, placed it next to the food processor, opened its lid, and emptied the drained beans into the food processor. *Ow. Ow. Ow. Ignore it. You're almost done. Now close the lid. Keep your right hand on top hard and hold it still, since you'll need to use your left finger to safely press the pulse button on and off. Here goes …*

*OH HOLY CRAP MY F***ING ARM'S ON FIRE! Okay, it's okay … Just rest a sec, breathe in, steel yourself, now press again – OH DEAR GOD IT HURTS LIKE HELL …*

And just like that, I'd made my little girl her first puréed veggies!

"You did great, Cathy."

"Thanks," I gasped, still trying to shake out my spastic arm and relax the raging pins and needles while I robot-walked to the cutlery drawer to get a big spoon. I picked up the spoon with my left hand; my right arm needed a rest, but I couldn't stop now. I had to finish this.

My wrist didn't have quite enough smooth circular movement to dig out a small scoop of puréed beans and then tap it cleanly into each section of the ice cube tray without me unleashing the spoon and making a goop-mess on the floor, so I quickly decided to scoop and tap with my left hand, and used my fatigued right fingers to keep the tray steady. Somehow, I managed to empty the bowl and fill 10 sections. My head was starting to pound like a 10-pin bowling ball hitting strike after strike … this had been a lot harder and taken longer than I expected, and there was still clean-up …

"I don't think Jean-Pierre will mind if I just rinse out the pot and the bowl of the food processor and leave it in the sink to dry. That's how we usually do it anyway," I said.

Sandra nodded. "You did really well today, Cathy. How do you feel?"

I turned around from the sink, smiling, dishes all rinsed, drying my hands on the tea towel, and leaned against the counter.

"I'm happy, but I'm just exhausted. And the headache's back."

"Well, that's to be expected," she assured me. "You're trying to retrain your body to do something new at the same time your injured brain is struggling to right itself, and it can be just plain exhausting."

"I'll say."

"One thing I try to encourage people to do down the road, like once you're home for good, is try to rest BEFORE you get tired. I know this will be a huge challenge for you as a first-time mother, but you have to try not to let yourself overdo it."

I nodded soberly. I felt myself fighting back tears.

"I'll call a cab now," Sandra said. "And there's just one more thing left for you to finish before we go get our coats on."

Bemused, I looked around, spotted the tray of puréed beans still on the counter. We both burst out laughing.

"Yeah, I guess it would help if I put it in the freezer!"

* * *

Slumped in the taxi after the horrendous task of fastening my seat belt, random thoughts ricocheted through my mind on the way back to Saint-Vincent's that Tuesday afternoon. Only three more days till my first weekend visit! I had successfully prepared baby food. This was very, very good … actually a huge step forward – being able to physically achieve a task independently, despite the insistent angry racket in my body. But ugh, how I hated car rides now; every little bump in the road assaulted me, making me seize and sting. But everything would be okay, I told myself; I just had to make it back to my bed and crash till it was time to drag myself into the hallway for supper.

5

Home on Weekends

After escaping his office on Friday around 4 p.m., Jean-Pierre blasted into my room with a wheelchair as if he was racing to catch a flight. He radiated agitation.

He gave me a peck and a quick "hi" and was about to help pull me off the bed as I put my penmanship exercises away. "I've got the car parked at the main entrance," he chirped. "Is your bag ready?"

I nodded and pointed to the closet. He threw my coat towards me. "You can put my bag on top of me once I'm in the chair," I said. "Are the brakes on?"

"What? Oh shit, yeah." He scrambled back to the chair and fumbled with the metal brake handles over each wheel. "There we go."

With deliberation, I sat and flipped the left footrest down into its proper position, but after just a little unsuccessful dithering with the right side, JP reached down, grasped my right ankle and put it in the right spot.

"Ow! You shouldn't do that for me," I complained, as he whirled me around and zoomed us into the hallway, making me feel as if I was on the Tilt-a-Whirl at the Ottawa Exhibition.

"I need all the practice I can get."

"Well, I don't want to keep the car out front any longer than we have to, and I don't want to keep Deb waiting too long."

Sandi Millar smiled as we flew past the nursing station. "Enjoy your weekend!" I waved a quick thanks.

When we got to the car, I began to give him instructions. "Okay, bring the chair up behind the front seat door. That's it. Now put the brakes back on the wheelchair, and you can open that friggin' heavy door for me." (It was a two-door 1981 Pontiac LeMans.) "Good. Yeah, put the bag in the back. Now I'm going to stand up. Yes. Thanks. Okay, just stay close while I get in - OW! NO! DON'T TOUCH MY RIGHT SIDE! I DON'T KNOW WHERE YOU ARE! I MIGHT JERK AND PULL YOU DOWN!"

His eyes widened, and his brow furrowed in dismay at my outburst. I plopped down into the passenger seat with a heavy sigh, and he hurried back into the lobby to return the chair. Whew! Transferring to and from the car took so much concentration and extra balancing; it was so tiring. I also noticed the drop down to get into the passenger seat was much farther compared to the taxi I rode in with Sandra Hobson just the other day.

"Sorry for shouting," I murmured, when he returned. "Still getting used to myself."

He nodded and forced a sad smile, closed my door and got in. "Yeah, me too." He watched me struggling with the seatbelt. I had to look far over and down to the right to see where I had to insert the buckle after losing my grip on it a couple of times.

"Need help with that?"

"No thanks." We both smiled when the buckle finally clicked.

"Thought I'd take the Rockcliffe Parkway home instead of stop-and-go on the Queensway at this hour."

"Oh, that's a good idea," I said. "Riding in the car's still pretty tough."

So off we went. Jean-Pierre is by far more talented behind the wheel than I am, but he has a heavy foot, and next to no patience with the other 90 per cent of the "stupid idiots" on the road. He tends to dart around the slower impediments, charge through yellow lights or slam the brakes upon deciding that the risk is too great. Fortunately though, he is a superb negotiator with the police. While having earned enough demerit points to risk mandatory road-rules refresher classes, he has also talked himself out of receiving at least three tickets. Once, he was pulled over by an undercover cop who had passed him on an entrance ramp to Highway 417 after an Ottawa Senators hockey game, because JP gave him his middle finger.

"Do you always give police the finger?" the officer asked.

"I didn't know you were a cop! You passed me on the ramp! I thought you were just another asshole!"

Anyway, the rush-hour trip through the downtown core to reach the Rockcliffe Parkway was exceedingly stop-and-go for me, despite JP's earnest efforts to behave. As darkness fell, the bright traffic lights assaulted me in crazy zigzags, hurting my eyes and building to a pounding crescendo. As we made the wide, zooming left turn from Rideau past the Conference Centre and around the Chateau Laurier to Sussex Drive, I put my head down, closed my eyes, and massaged them gently.

"Headache?"

"Oh ya. I don't do well in cars anymore."

He reached over and caressed my thigh. "Poor you. Should get better once we're on the Parkway."

"Okay, but don't speed to get there."

He grinned. "Ha! You're not out of the hospital five minutes, and you're already nagging me."

We both chuckled while I kept my eyes shut.

Once on the Eastern Parkway, the majestic two-lane road passed the Official Residences of the Prime Minister and Governor General, then imperceptibly rose high through the tall trees, past embassies, up to and around the infamous rock cliff like a roller coaster, hundreds of feet above the Ottawa River. Huge, yellowish icicles coated the northeast side of the tall crag, while round white antique light bulbs atop cast-iron lamp posts glowed along the river railing. That night, these stunning old-fashioned street lights assaulted me with a rapid succession of painful flashes, until finally, the cliff mercifully levelled off to flatter, safer ground flanking the river, and after we passed the Rockcliffe Boat House, the rapid glaring finally faded. With a shudder, I welcomed the darkness. For me, one of Ottawa's most awe-inspiring scenic drives had morphed into a ridiculous scene from the *Rocky Horror Picture Show.* It was my first preview of a later diagnosis related to my damaged thalamus: photophobia – a blinding sensitivity to bright lights.

Some 10 minutes later, we arrived at Debra Laxton's townhouse in our Pineview neighbourhood.

The Laxtons lived walking distance from our townhouse, but I had never set foot in this particular project before. Nor did I, that night. I wasn't up for any "meet and greet your baby's caregiver," and I was too exhausted to feel guilty about it. All I could think about was making it home, and waiting for my girl to appear in JP's arms. I watched him hurry across the parking lot, ring the doorbell, and rush in. No polite waves from the doorway this evening.

Less than a minute passed before the door opened, and there she was, all bundled up in her portable car seat, or the "Bub," as that particular model was often called, stoically brought towards me by her devoted Poppa Hen.

"Ahh, allô ma petite … I wish I could see you right now," I cooed, as JP turned the Bub around backwards to correctly fasten her into the rear seat, and he quickly shut the door, so she wouldn't get a chill.

"There!" He jumped into the front seat, smiling. He looked exhausted.

"Yes … home, James," I joked, feigning a prissy British accent.

Before I knew it, we were pulling into the driveway.

"I'll bring her inside, then I'll come get you, okay?"

"Sounds good."

I watched him hurry inside, and overwhelmed by his love for her, my sad heart warmed a little. Quick as he was, he was back in a flash, and opened my door.

"Ready?"

"Yup." I raised my right leg, swivelled myself 90 degrees with my left, positioned my legs on the snowy asphalt, and then stood, and he was already going for my right arm to support me.

"No, no, hon. I might pull you down … "

"No you won't."

"NO! Don't grab me there! I need to get free of the door on my own, and then you take my LEFT arm, okay?"

Thank God I didn't have aphasia; at least I could keep a running commentary on what we had to deal with, especially since it was constantly changing.

The three of us were together now in the foyer, our little darling still waiting patiently on the floor in her Bub, puffed up in her snowsuit, with my stoic, heartbroken husband by her side. The real healing had now begun.

We put our arms around each other, and our kiss lingered in a way it had not since our ordeal began.

"Welcome home," he whispered. "I love you."

"I love you, too. So glad to be back." I grinned. "You'll probably be relieved to get me back to Saint-Vincent's on Sunday, though."

We took our coats off. "Let's get you two settled in the living room. The car ride was hard on you, wasn't it?"

"Yeah, first time travelling at night. The lights really bothered me."

As I mentioned, I was later diagnosed with photophobia, an extreme sensitivity to bright light. Again, this was due to the thalamic damage from the stroke, which affected the functioning of all my sensations, and further increased by the side-effects of a couple of essential brain-calming medications. Now, all day, I wear prescription sunglasses with a slight clearness at the bottom of the bifocals for reading, and on a bright, sunny or headachy day, I have darker clip-ons to put on top of the sunglasses.

Our sweet baby girl gurgled at us, flailing her arms in her Bub. I smiled at her and cooed, "Ooh, our petite bébé needs to be freed, doesn't she?"

"Go get comfy on the couch, and I'll bring her to you."

I stayed to watch him carefully unbuckle her, unzip her snowsuit, extricate her chubby little arms and legs, and lift her up into his arms with a smile. I came over and tickled her chin. Her little mouth turned upwards, her eyes big and staring, full of wonder, right into mine.

"Wow, you're a pro," I said softly. "She looks so content."

"Lotsa practice. Come on, let's get you two settled. She'll probably be ready for her bottle pretty soon."

The three of us travelled the bumpy, orange shag hallway together, well on our way to rebooting our lives.

At least today, anyway.

I sat down on the hideous black-and-white plaid loveseat I bought for my first apartment. There were a few cushions that I propped under my left arm, and JP settled her into its crook. I slowly jerked my right arm here and there, in an effort to find the safest position I could hold for the longest period of time. I nodded, and JP placed her in my arms for real this time, at home.

Eyes wide, she stared into my tearful eyes, my sad smile. She knew I was her Mom, but I felt different to her now. Something big had changed me, and she wasn't sure what to make of it. I teared up and kissed her forehead.

"Oh, my sweetie," I murmured. "I will do everything I can to come back to you." Jean-Pierre sat down beside me and put his arms around us. I jerked. *Burn burn burn. Fuck off, burning.*

"How's it going?"

"Good," I lied.

"How 'bout I warm up a bottle and we can see how that goes?"

"Sure. We'd like that."

He sprang off the couch. He needed to keep busy. I heard the fridge door and cupboards opening and closing … it was so weird to hear him thrashing about in the kitchen, but I was so happy just to gaze at my little girl, concentrating on keeping my gridlock hold on her, watching her watching me.

"Good timing," I said, when he appeared with a perfectly warmed bottle of formula. "She was just starting to squirm."

"Want me to help you put this in your hand?"

I nodded. "Just turn it upside down for me and then I'll try to grab it and position it myself."

On our first attempt, the bottle slipped out of her mouth and fell onto the carpet. Her eyes, incredulous, followed its path, and she squawked, circling her arms impatiently. She had no intention of missing out on a good bottle.

I giggled. "Sorry, honey. We gotta clean up that nipple now." JP dutifully retrieved the bottle and rinsed it off. When he came back, I asked him to spot us first because her wriggling had weakened my hold on her and I felt unstable. I managed to better reposition us against the arm of the couch, then gripped the bottle as tightly as I could and prayed that I would not shove it up a nostril or into her eye.

She latched on immediately though, and drank heartily. JP smiled, watching. About a minute later though, she squeezed her eyes together and coughed, and I struggled to get her more upright so I could pat her back. The bottle dropped on the floor again, and my baby stared at me, confused. I continued fussing to try to secure her, and just like her Mommy, she started to fuss. Again, Mr. Mom leapt to retrieve the errant bottle.

"Houston, we have a problem," I said. "She's slipping."

He swept her away from me, held her in one arm and with the bottle in the other, brought her into the kitchen, and rinsed off the bottle. I got myself up from the loveseat and bent over at the waist, trying to shake out the tension in my exhausted arms, trying to convince myself that I should be thrilled. I fed my baby girl (if only for a minute)! That was progress, wasn't it? I looked outside at the darkness, at her highchair at the head of our teak dining room table, at the piano on my left, and sat back down. I would not break down. Not yet.

He came out of the kitchen, holding and feeding her. "Hey," he said softly, sitting in the maroon velour tub chair. "You need to rest. You'd said the ride was tough."

Oh yeah, seems like eons ago. I nodded, put a cushion behind my head, and lay back, legs hanging over the arm of the loveseat.

"Guess what I'm making for supper tonight?" There was excitement in his voice.

"What? Just tell me."

"How does spaghetti carbonara sound?"

"Yum. Good."

I closed my eyes. *Hmm … this should be interesting. At least he's watched me make it. Whisk an egg in a bowl, whisk in with some cream, grated parmesan, a bit of chili peppers; then add piping hot al dente spaghetti, drained but not rinsed; then put it into the bowl along with sauteed little pieces of bacon, and … presto!*

My thoughts travelled back to the first time we tried this delicacy at La Ripaille, an enchanting restaurant in old-town Québec City, before we married. Jean-Pierre had taken on a five-month acting assignment at a Transport Canada location right on the St. Lawrence River in the Port of Québec, and we spent a few romantic weekends together. It was so sweet of him to think of preparing something to remind us of those carefree, happier days …

I roused myself to hear him thrashing around in the kitchen again. My charge was right next to me on the floor, safely strapped in her Bub, sucking on a soother, looking calm and content.

"Allô, ma petite fille. Whatcha doin' down there?"

Jean-Pierre rushed over, looking stressed. "Supper will be ready soon. Can you make your way to the table? I'll get her installed in the high chair."

"Okay, hon. I'll do her bib."

Before I was fully standing, he'd already swung her over like a roller coaster to her maple throne. She smiled, vocalized and kicked her legs about, playfully resisting his forceful efforts to shove them through the appropriate spaces. Eventually though, Poppa Hen prevailed.

"Can I set the table?"

"Sure. I'll be bringing out some beans, pablum and the rest of her bottle. Wanna feed her?"

"Yes, yes!"

From there, things deteriorated rapidly. Somehow, her cute all-in-one food dish got knocked to the floor, then by the time Mr. Mom had cleaned up that disaster and started over, he discovered his hot spaghetti sitting in the raw egg mixture, untossed and cold.

"AW SHIT … "

He stared at the bowl, scowled, put his head down, and began swearing a blue streak –

"STOP IT! JUST STOP!"

Shocked by our raised voices, our baby girl crinkled her mouth, about to release a sob.

"Oh, I'm so sorry, my sweetie." I gently stroked her soft blond hair and felt relief that this calmed her.

"Hey, it's no big deal, hon." I reassured him. "Just stir it together and zap it in the microwave once or twice, and it'll be fine. We'll just pretend it's an Italian omelet."

With a tired sigh, he did as he was told. "I just wanted to do something special for you, your first time back … "

"I know, hon." He was trying so hard, and I felt so bad for him.

Before the stroke, I handled all the chef duties. His own cooking experience from his six months living solo came mainly from a seven-block stretch on Montreal Road, not far from where he grew up on rue Montfort in Vanier: Eastview Pizza's savoury Lebanese pizza, egg rolls from Wings, or coke and jukebox tunes at Blue Sky, the Midnight BBQ, or the always-crowded El Matador. He also made his sister Céline's deadly good recipe of chicken fried rice with sausage, sauteed in an electric frying pan.

I, on the other hand, inherited a few of my Mom's "Mennonite health-food nut" tendencies, so we enjoyed plenty of opportunities to exercise our differences of opinion on the food-prep front.

We three ate our tasty mush, pretty much in silence, save for a giggle or two when I gave my girl a few mashed-up pieces of overcooked eggy noodles to play with. She made a happy mess stuffing the morsels into her mouth, making her sulking Poppa Hen break into unexpected laughter.

She was our glue. She kept us focussed on getting better, for her.

* * *

Our TV was in the finished basement, but we didn't go down that first night. Our only goal was for me to make it upstairs, and help change her diaper, get her into jammies and tuck her away safely in her crib.

Climbing the stairs went a lot better than expected. JP had never seen me do stairs before, so he was understandably apprehensive.

I managed not to blurt out "ow ow ow" as my right hand gripped the wooden railing, mainly because wood felt far less painful than the cold metal rail at Saint-Vincent's. The rise of each step was also a bit lower than the hospital's stairwell and therefore, much less onerous for lifting the legs. However, the thick carpeting on our stairs required heightened concentration to make sure the right foot was safely placed. Just like my physiotherapist Kathy Eyre, Jean-Pierre was at my back, one step behind me, just in case I faltered.

Only the last step, which had a bigger carpet lip and less support from the end of the railing, required me to expel a final "oomph!," but I had made it onto the landing on the second floor by myself, and fairly quickly, too!

"Wow," JP said from the stairs. "I'm impressed."

"Yeah. Gotta love Saint-Vincent Boot Camp."

Upstairs, the main bathroom, directly across from our daughter's room on the southwest corner, provided a long, wide counter to the right of the sink, which was a perfect fit for her on her changing mat. The wall-to-wall vanity mirror also provided a complete view of her playfully kicking and grasping the air as she lay on her back, gaily awaiting the next new moves from her unpredictable parents.

I'm guarding her, making sure she doesn't fall off the counter. I know this place, but it's as if I've never been here before, like I don't know what I can do, or how to try to do it. Oh well, it's all good, we all seem to have gotten over being so upset at suppertime. Ahh, Jean-Pierre has now returned with a fresh nappy and a comfy jammy ...

"Let me do it," I insisted. With JP standing beside me, I pulled off her sleeves, and then the footed legs of her onesie; then with my left hand, I grasped her two legs together and lifted her bottom up, and JP helped remove the rest of the onesie from underneath her.

Then off came her diaper, using the same technique. JP did not need to intervene, except for putting it in the diaper pail. He passed me a small terry cloth and I cleaned and dried her off, noticing a small area of diaper rash on her inner thigh. Keeping her stable with my left hand, I rattled the top drawer open with my right, and spied the flat canister of diaper rash cream. *Aha, pay dirt!* I tried to pick it up, but it fell onto the floor with a nasty clang and started rolling away. Before I had a chance to curse, Mr. Quick and Efficient had already retrieved it and removed its lid for me.

"Oh, thanks, hon."

"Where would you like it?"

"Right next to the mirror; that way she can't kick it off." I switched gears, steadying her with my right hand and dabbing her rash with my left. *Safety Rule Number 161: Limit experimentation with fine motor skills when sensitive body parts are involved.*

I lifted her legs again; JP passed me the fresh diaper, and I managed to place it well enough under her bottom, and fasten her up satisfactorily, even though the taping job was markedly crooked. The learning curve of figuring out new ways to do everyday things made me feel like a young child myself.

"There you go, ma petite!" I blew my lips on her belly, making a fluttering farty sound, and she giggled. My confidence soared, and that's when I knew everything was going to be okay. She was still squirming with delight, so I let Jean-Pierre take over most of the pyjama dressing. I was spent from the intense concentration.

"How's it going with the sandbag?"

"Ahh, it's okay for weight training, but it sags all over the place."

"Not like a real human 'bean,' eh?"

I shook my head. "Not at all."

"How 'bout I put her in your arms and we can cross the hall together to her crib?" I hesitated. "I'll take her from you to put her in the crib, then you can cover her with her blankie," he said, trying to reassure me and cover up his own unease.

For the second time that day, I experienced the deep joy of my loving husband surrendering our precious daughter to me, and even with him stepping backwards with his arms under mine in case I faltered, my left arm became her anchor, with my right arm a squawking, clumsy but willing learner. Her eyes moved back and forth at us.

Hmmm, she's watching us do more new things. I'm back, but I'm very nervous carrying her … but JP's guarding us and minding us closely … and he doesn't look as grim right now. I like this …

I kissed her warm forehead and put her face against mine for a little while, then Poppa Hen took her from me and carefully laid her down. Then we hugged. I got her blankie and tucked her in. *Everything is so different now. I'm never exactly sure how to do anything yet … and I'm so afraid of hurting her. I need to be so careful … oh, ha ha, you love your soother, don't you, my sweetie … Mommy and Daddy say … kissy kissy … nighty night …*

✳ ✳ ✳

Jean-Pierre stayed with me while I sat on the edge of our waterbed, got undressed and put my own flannels on. He reached towards me, always trying to make things easier, but I shook my head, mentally pushing him away.

"No," I insisted. "I need to be able to do everything by myself. I'll never make it if you don't let me figure it out." JP looked hurt; he took my rebuke personally. "It's not you; it's me," I tried to explain, as I fumbled with the buttons on the shirt. JP looked like he was going to cry.

"I can't stand to watch you struggle," he murmured, looking away.

"Well maybe tomorrow morning, I'll try just leaving the buttons done up when I take it off, so that next time I can just pull it over my head and then slip my arms through the sleeves," I offered.

He helped me get into our queen-size waterbed. I closed my eyes, smiling. "Ah, it feels so nice, being back with you in our own bed," I murmured.

With my eyes still closed, he grasped my right hand, and we were both shocked by the involuntary jerk that shuddered through me.

"Sorry!"

"No – I'M sorry! Didn't see you coming!" I forced a chuckle to make him smile.

"I'll let you get settled while I tidy up a bit downstairs, and then I think I'll take a little break," he said softly.

"Kay. See you."

After we kissed and he left, I let the fluid surround me, pleasantly amazed at how great it felt. With the water mattress, there were almost no pressure points activating the abnormal burning stinging response to touch on my right side, and whenever I moved, the water shifted with me with a few comforting ripples, maintaining consistent and comforting pressure. That was the beginning of my discovery over many years that by applying consistent coverage on my affected side, like long sleeves and a scarf around the prickly side of my neck, it helped reduce jerky, spastic reactions from breezes, cold, fatigue, muscular pain and later, menopausal hot flashes. Heck, now I often go out wearing my sweaters with the right arm in its sleeve and the left sleeve wrapped around my neck like a scarf. Now that I'm in my sixties, and I don't care as much how ridiculous I might appear to others.

I am also grateful for the hipsters who now wear high-top sneakers with a dress. Smart and supportively casual – without feeling dowdy about no heels! I got myself some beautifully comfortable, grey-suede high tops designed in Brazil, and I wore them every day and night when my girl and I enjoyed a marvellous Mom-and-daughter-only week in Holguin, Cuba, in February 2020. I also brought super-supportive laced-up water shoes and my own snorkel mask for the beautiful coral reef the resort was nestled on. We made it back to Canada just before the first COVID-19 pandemic lockdown began. The only face masks we saw were on a few Holguin airport staff. I will never forget how fortunate we were to share that intimate time together in such a wondrous place before the world as we knew it changed forever.

* * *

I continued to make excellent progress at Saint-Vincent Hospital with the weekend home visits, and shortly before my discharge in mid-March, with continued outpatient physiotherapy twice a week, I had one last safety move I needed to master: getting in and out of the bathtub.

Getting in is pretty routine; left hand against the wall (or on the grab bar, 30 years later), then left foot over and in, quickly followed by the right, over and in, then ease yourself down, balancing with both hands firmly on the edge of the tub. Check.

Getting out is the biggest challenge. From the sitting position, turn your upper body around to the left, so that you are facing the back of the tub, and using your left arm as the stabilizer, turn your lower body over so that you are on hands and knees, just like a doggie. (Arf!) Okay, good. Now, you have to be super careful here. Survey yourself. How is your right leg positioned? Make sure that big toe is far enough away from the edge of the giant bath mat, so that it won't get caught underneath while you're in the process of sliding the leg forward to stand up … now, once you feel completely stable, lift your left hand up to the tub edge and put your right hand against the wall. OK now, do you feel balanced? Good, now slide your right leg wonkily forward, watch the foot like a hawk as it struggles to place itself as flat as it can on the bath mat, again making sure the big toe doesn't get caught. Then, when the knee is safely right-angled with the foot on the floor, push up your left leg to join with the right, lean over to bring the right hand to rest on the tub edge with the left, place the right leg over to the left, and as soon as it's secure, place all your weight on the hands and then lift the left leg over the tub, plant it on the secured rug, then bring the right leg up and over, then let go of the tub and rise to a standing position.

Then I would dry myself off and go lie down because the whole process of getting out of the tub wore me out to the bone.

6

Healing for Good

After seven weeks at Saint-Vincent Hospital, I no longer needed Xanax to calm my anxiety, and everyone agreed that I would be released from their wonderful care and support – except for Tuesdays and Thursdays, when I would return for outpatient physiotherapy. Since I was not yet allowed to drive, and JP needed to stay at the office, I took Para Transpo, the City of Ottawa's much-maligned transportation service for people with disabilities. You were required to call the day before to arrange a pick-up. For medical appointments, Para Transpo was fairly punctual. But they were god-awful for trips that were considered "non-priority." I learned this by waiting two-and-a-half hours for a drive from the hospital to St. Laurent Shopping Centre. So much for my efforts to enjoy a "fun" afternoon at a mall.

In the beginning, Debra took care of our daughter on those

two days per week that I went to physiotherapy. As well, every Friday for the first few weeks was a "free" day for me to rest up and experiment with my ever-improving physical skills and tolerance levels. I would test my ability to perform everyday tasks in my own new "senseless" way, at home, all by myself and free of distractions. Like making the bed, dressing myself, holding a broom to sweep the floor, going for a short walk or making a recipe. The fatigue and burning from my weakened right side, particularly in my neck and arm, combined with the constant need to figure out how to do everything before starting to do it, felt endless, onerous and discouraging.

The Mondays and Wednesdays I had my sweet pea all to myself from 6:30 a.m. to 4 p.m. were a blur for both of us. I could lift her out of her high chair now and make it to the couch or her playpen, but I couldn't carry her upstairs after breakfast, at first. We stayed in the living room most of the day; she napped in her playpen while I crashed next to her on the couch.

It's interesting that she never crawled. As well-meaning but isolated parents, we didn't know about the importance of "tummy time," so she always rotated around and around on her little rear end. Just before her first birthday, she grabbed onto the coffee table, stood up and started walking. Looking back at her early photos, her face was often a bit too serious. That breaks my heart.

Our daughter continued to be in Debra's care for a few years. I felt so much guilt on the days I was at home by myself, without my daughter, knowing she was in someone else's care, less than a mile away. Debra was amazing though; she was very quiet, steadfast, loving and so respectful – another angel sent to us. It was good for our little girl to be there too because she got to play and socialize with the other wee ones in a much more spontaneous, positive space.

Debra was strict too; she did not tolerate any bad behaviour from her minions. One day when JP arrived to pick up our little darling, who was about two at the time, Deb opened the door, and quickly slipped outside, her face, grave.

"Something happened today with your daughter that I need to talk to you about," she said tersely.

Jean-Pierre's eyes widened. "Oh? What happened?"

Deb lowered her eyes. "She punched David in the face."

"Jesus! How come?"

"I'm not sure. I think they were fighting over a toy."

"Oh dear … "

"Anyway, while David was crying, I separated them for a while, and I was very firm with her. I told her what she did was wrong, that she should never, ever hit other people, and that I will not tolerate that kind of behaviour here."

JP nodded emphatically. "Oh my, Debra. Thank you so much for setting her straight. We'll make it clear to her that if she ever does anything like that again, you will not take care of her anymore."

Debra nodded slowly, agreeing to his promise, and then she brought our shamed little She-Devil to her father. Much later, our daughter told us she put her fist in David's face because he stepped on and broke her yellow plastic briefcase, which held all her craft papers.

In bed that night, we held each other and tried not to laugh too hard.

* * *

Wherever we went, we always brought our munchkin with us and treated her as an equal participant in our team. Even as a baby, she never threw tantrums or made a scene in public.

Okay; it did happen once, at the Emerald Garden Chinese Restaurant downtown on Rideau Street.

One crisp, Arctic night after I'd been home full-time for about a month, JP and I had a serious craving for the Emerald Garden's succulent shrimp with pineapple and ginger, so we packed up our darling into her snowsuit and Bub seat and set off to indulge. We scored the last available table: a three-seater right across from the front entrance of the tiny, glass-fronted restaurant, so we kept her in her snowsuit and Bub to make sure she stayed toasty.

No fussing at all as our friendly waitress smiled and nodded at our beautiful little girl, then pleasantly acknowledged our favourite orders and hurried away.

However, when our food arrived, our little one launched into raging wails. She sounded like a fire truck barrelling towards a five-alarm fire. The other diners started to look increasingly disturbed.

Nothing would stop her wailing. We tried giving her a soother, which she spat out in disgust. Maybe she was too hot – Poppa Hen undid her snowsuit, cradled her and rubbed her back. That calmed our little girl a tad, but as soon as she was returned to her perch, she just screamed and screamed and screamed. JP checked her diaper, then bundled her up again and took her for a quick walk outside. A few minutes later, he returned, looking freaked out as she started screaming again, the instant they were back inside. By this time, dirty looks soured the faces of everyone.

"Here hon, give her to me. Pass me her bottle and chow down," I told him. "We gotta get out of here."

He gobbled frantically for a few minutes while she continued fussing, then took her from me, signalled for the bill and finished securing our disgruntled bundle of joy while I scarfed down what was left.

"You pay the bill, and I'll see you in the car," he told me as he left with our petite offender. Maybe she found the exotic smells of the food intolerable. Or maybe she was furious with us for not sharing with her. She hadn't peed or pooped either. We'll never know.

Our waitress politely completed the VISA transaction. I gave her an extra big tip.

"Next time, it'll be just the two of us," I promised. "Then we'll be able to take our time, and enjoy more of your delicious eastern coffee."

She smiled, nodded and unclasped her hands to wave goodbye as I struggled out of my chair.

* * *

It took us a few more years before we realized what eastern coffee really was.

Seated at the back of the Emerald Garden one night, we ordered eastern coffee after another delicious repast. Our server nodded, smiled and hurried over to a stall near the kitchen entrance, where we saw her rip open single-serve packets of Sanka decaffeinated, instant coffee! We couldn't stop laughing. What foolish foodies we were!

7

Getting My Driver's Licence Back

After a stroke, neurological or significant head injury, a physician is obligated to revoke the affected individual's legal right to operate a motor vehicle, until it can be determined that the person's condition is stable enough to undergo specific testing to assess whether they need assistive devices in order to drive safely. In my case, Dr. Clifford notified what is now known as the Ottawa Hospital Rehabilitation Centre, which manages driving rehabilitation, that I was now fit to undergo the diagnostic testing process. I was so looking forward to getting past this hurdle six months after the stroke, and finally being able to drive again!

The sun was high and bright as I entered the Royal Ottawa Rehabilitation Centre, as it was known back then, for the first and only time I would ever need to, I assumed. It was a bold, vibrant, beautiful place of caring and energetic support from health professionals for the "royally" disabled. The most immediately visible patients were those who had progressed to wheelchairs, particularly amputees of various extremities; yet they all looked surprisingly positive as they flitted up, down and around the huge, bright concourses angled in unconventional directions, taking elevators independently, giving it their all because they knew how lucky they were to have this opportunity to benefit from a second (or third, or fourth) chance to find new ways to rebuild their own lives.

These vibes humbled me as I made my way to find Driving Rehabilitation Services. Upon arrival, I was warmly greeted by occupational therapist Joe Pialunga. His smile was perpetual, exuding caring and kindness.

"Welcome! You must be Cathy," he said, extending his hand to shake mine.

Instinctively, my stronger left hand rose to reciprocate, but then froze as I realized I could not shake hands with my left if the initiator offered their right.

"Oops – sorry!" I blurted, embarrassed. Light chuckles amid shifting hands and assurances of "no worries" followed, but I finally insisted on shaking with my right hand, with the stinging included, since most people are right-handed.

"You look like you're doing really well," said Joe. He extended his arms across the large room to direct me to the car driving simulator, and I got into the driver's seat. "Okay, good. Now, we'll slide you a bit closer to the pedals. Is that better?"

I watched my right foot touch the gas pedal, and then found

the brake. "Yes, that's good."

"All right then, today we're going to be assessing your peripheral vision field cut and your right foot's ability to react and shift from the gas to the brake pedals."

"Good, let's do it!" I was going to ace this.

He pressed a few buttons on the console of the large viewing screen, and a crude street map appeared. I interpreted the large flashing dot to be my car, and another grid labelled "kph" would tell me how fast I would be travelling in kilometres. He explained that I would be receiving different commands to "turn left" or "'take McPherson Road," but at any time, a red light could flash and require me to hit the brakes.

At first it seemed fairly straightforward. Though I felt like I was forcing my concentration and slamming my foot all the time, my responses seemed immediate enough. But as the test wore on, I could only smash down on the brakes with half of my foot or just the end of it because I had to keep my eyes focussed strictly on the road for the other cars, stop signs or a darting child, and not on my foot. Once, my foot unexpectedly missed the brake completely, but I seemed to relocate it immediately. You're just rusty. With practice, you'll improve …

When the test finally ended, relief poured out of me. I felt like I'd been holding my breath the whole time, but I had survived. It had felt gruelling, though.

Joe nodded at me from his analysis station with a warm smile. "Thanks Cathy. Just bear with me for a few minutes while I put the results together."

I nodded, hoping I did not appear too anxious, but I could not stop staring at his calm, intent profile, watching his every move: his brown eyes glued to the screen, then quickly dropping down to the keyboard as his fingers tapped away in short bursts.

"Okay," he said softly, and he finally came back over. "The good news is that you will be able to drive a car again without any retraining, but you will need to use a left-foot gas pedal."

I stared at him, dumbstruck.

"Really?"

"I'm afraid so," he said, but his expression was cheerful. "With your high spasticity and lack of sensation in that right foot, your safety is compromised. There's no getting around that."

"Okay. I get it."

His million-dollar smile of optimism continued. "We'll still schedule you for a driver's test here at the Rehab Centre, and the car will be equipped with a left-foot gas pedal that just flips down to use it. I also want to reassure you that the testers at the Rehab Centre are extremely considerate, and they won't be asking you to do things like parallel park. You'll be issued a permanent disabled driver permit."

I nodded, soaking in the totally unexpected news, and dreading JP's angst at having another complication thrown on top of our already overflowing must-do list.

"Here," he said, "I have a left-foot gas pedal attachment I can show you." He left me floating in my state of shock for a few seconds while he bounded off to retrieve the device. Still smiling, he showed me the shiny aluminum contraption: a pedal with a stabilizing grid and a long bar designed to extend across the floor and attach to the functioning gas pedal.

"See? To use it, you just flip it down like this, and then you're good to go."

"Hmmm. That's not so bad."

"No it's not," he agreed, his aura so reassuring and inspiring. "It'll feel rather strange at first, but you'll quickly get used to it."

"Okay, so how do I get one?"

"We have them available here, and this is sufficient for the test, but they're not that durable, so you might want to consider finding a mechanic who can actually install another gas pedal on the left side of the car."

Finding an able and willing mechanic in 1984 was not easy, though. There were very few who had even heard of doing such a thing, let alone having any experience actually doing it. Most didn't want to even look at a job like that, since every model of every car of every year can be different, and they didn't feel comfortable hacking up a vehicle only to discover they were mistaken in what they thought would work.

Eventually we found Dave, owner of Bayview Motors, who had done some similar jobs for drivers with disabilities. However, Dave spent an even longer amount of time obtaining a compatible gas pedal that would fit into where it had to go.

By the time the car was ready in early September, I was raring to go. I had already passed my road test at the Rehab Centre in June.

JP picked up the car on a Saturday, and that afternoon, I insisted on taking the car out. By myself. I couldn't get distracted or made more nervous by anyone else interrupting my impaired senses – I had to get used to my own new, counterintuitive way of driving, first. I needed to be particularly prudent with my right-sided visual field cut and always turn my head farther to the right, to make sure I didn't miss anything important. I also needed a while to get used to speeding up and slowing down from the left side.

So off I went, on a long, slow, glorious drive that eventually meandered through Beechwood Cemetery, the resting place of past Prime Ministers, Canada's military heroes and scores of other local and national notables, with the road through the cemetery circling around hills of majestic maples and rapturous gardens. It made me feel so happy that I was still alive.

It's not yet time for me to rest here, though.

Hmmm ... now you don't want to get so exhausted that you make a mistake ... remember, you gotta pace yourself, make it back home before you get too tired ...

So I turned our Pontiac LeMans around and headed home.

Everything went just fine. I pulled into the driveway, and ...

BLAAAAAMMMM!!!

WTF? I just slammed into the garage door!!

Aww, shit ... I got the gas and the brake mixed up ...

Shaken from his nap, Jean-Pierre exploded out the front door, gawked at the crumpled garage door, then rushed over to me, still at the wheel, shaking my head, my hand on my forehead.

He opened my door. "My God, what happened? Are you okay?"

"Yeah, yeah," I muttered, disgusted with my ineptitude. "I'm so sorry ... I was doing just fine, but then I got the pedals mixed up at the very end."

"Shit … you really did a number on the door!"

I got out and looked around. "Well, at least the car doesn't have a scratch. That's good."

"I'll call Mr. Hovi. He'll replace it for us." Mr. Hovi was our condo's maintenance guy, our outdoor fixer-upper, according to our condo board's manifesto of uniformity.

"That'll probably cost us a few hundred bucks," I murmured to JP, as he shouldered me into our unit.

The ever-prompt Mr. Hovi replaced our garage door the following week. Turns out we were never charged a penny. Either the condo board felt sorry for us, or perhaps they decided to list it as a "miscellaneous maintenance" expense.

8

Sterilization

In addition to the gruelling everyday challenges that came from emerging from "zombie state" and continuing to improve as a Mommy, bigger issues plagued us. For some time, we had been requesting a consultation with the Ottawa General Hospital's Chief Neurologist, Dr. Nelson; Jean-Pierre was convinced that my toke or two of cannabis was the major cause of the stroke, but more importantly, we also wanted Dr. Nelson's medical opinion about whether it would be safe for me to get pregnant again. We had always wanted to have two children, at least before the stroke.

Finally, very late one afternoon, we met with Dr. Nelson and the kindly Dr. Skinner, his second in command. As to cannabis causing the stroke, their answer was a definitive "no." It was a blood clot.

As to another pregnancy, he hummed and hawed. JP finally

said, "Look, if she was your wife, would you want her to get pregnant again?"

His eyes dropped and he shook his head. "No, I wouldn't."

While we were not surprised with his assessment, we needed a second opinion on such a life-altering decision from my obstetrician, who would be more of an expert on confirming the risks of another stroke resulting from a subsequent pregnancy.

So the next stop for me was Dr. Puddicombe, who had delivered my baby vaginally after I refused his last-minute terse advice to have a cesarean, which forced him to stitch me up like a soldier on the battlefield after I ripped apart. I sincerely regret not having listened to him.

I was ushered into his dark, comfortable office, and he stood up from behind his large, ornately carved wooden desk, smiled and shook my hand.

"It's so good to see you again, Cathy," he said, smiling warmly. "Please, have a seat. How are you doing?"

"Much better, thanks." I fumbled to sit down and get comfortable. "It's certainly not easy, but it's so much better now that I'm back home."

"I'm so glad to hear that," he said, sitting down and leaning forward from the giant desk. "So, how can I help you today?"

"Well, I just wanted your opinion on whether you think it would be safe for me to ever get pregnant again."

He didn't answer right away, and slowly blew out some air from pursed lips. "Well … pregnancy puts more stress on the cardiovascular system than just about anything else, and given your history, I would have to say I would definitely not recommend it. If I were you, Cathy, I would be happy that you have one healthy little girl and that you are still here with us."

I nodded soberly. "You know, I'm really glad you're telling me this because I am terrified of getting pregnant again," I admitted. "JP and I are just trying to come to terms with everything and considering other possibilities like adoption, so at least we won't feel guilty about not trying anymore … "

"Oh, I am SO relieved," he said with a smile, closing his eyes and shaking his head. "I thought you were here to tell me you wanted to have another baby."

* * *

It didn't take much more pondering for us to decide that given all the new wrenches thrown into our daily lives managing my disabilities, and the fact that even with the best intentions, adoptions were a crapshoot in terms of knowing less about what kinds of issues you could end up coping with, we decided we were quite content being parents of our beautiful only child.

Since it was less than a year after my stroke, and pregnancy would be a danger to me, we sought out a urologist who could perform a reversible vasectomy on Jean-Pierre, in the event that I were to suddenly pass away. Jean-Pierre was still a young man, and I didn't want to saddle him with sterility if I was to suddenly die or become a vegetable; I wanted him to find another life partner with whom he could share the joys of bringing a new person into the world, a step-sibling for our little girl.

When we went to see Dr. Shapiro, who was considered to be

an expert in reversible vasectomies, he grilled us about our intentions. He sat there, deadpan, listening to us explain our rationale and pour out our wishes for each other, offering a brief nod here and there.

"Oh yeah," I added nervously, after pouring out our hearts, "and a vasectomy would be far less invasive for him than for me to undergo a tubal 'litigation' … "

Dr. Shapiro burst out laughing. "You mean – ha ha ha! – a tubal LIGATION!"

We all roared. No, I wouldn't be taking my ovaries to the Supreme Court anytime soon …

When Jean-Pierre returned for the clipping of his vas deferens, he asked Dr. Shapiro how soon it would be before he could safely have intercourse again.

"Well, at least wait till you get home," he replied, deadpan.

9

Grocery Shopping Traumas

Though I was off the anxiety meds, completing certain every-day tasks still filled me with dread, including any kind of shopping. I quickly learned that latching on to a shopping cart was always step number one, even if I needed just one or two things. It anchored me, and I wouldn't have to worry about how to carry anything until checking out. Often, my neck, arm and hand unexpectedly pulsed with raw stinging pain, be it from a draft, fatigue or contact with anything metallic. A stinging tin can of tuna would make me forget what I was looking for, even if I carried a list. Cold metal was always brutal. I had to remind myself not to put anything important in my right pocket either. I'd forget it was there because I had no sense of where it was against my body. I'd even forget what I was holding in my right hand, and often ended up misplacing so many things. When too many things disturbed me all at once, I'd feel terror, a sense that I was losing control. *Will I be able to do this? What if I can't finish? What if I can't follow through after I've paid … can I make it back to the car? Relax, the cart is your walker … but what if I need to sit down, or lie down? I must make sure nobody bumps me because they have no idea how much I'm struggling. What if someone knocks me over?*

The first time I walked into the grocery store alone, I found myself panting from anxiety, so I pulled the cart over to a quiet corner, closed my eyes and forced deep, slow breaths, in and out, in and out …

Look, Cath, this is a non-negotiable, essential activity. You must do this. Go beyond the burning … all this walking, pushing, stretching and grasping will help you get stronger … and when you get home, you can have a big-ass lie-down. It won't be a nap, since you never really sleep till the bedtime meds, but …

* * *

One awful afternoon, on one of my first solo "excursions" to the grocery store, I turned the corner into the cereal aisle and nearly rammed my cart into our caregiver Debra. In her cart sat my darling daughter with little David.

We were both tongue-tied with discomfort. Debra was not a woman of many words, and I found it devastating to suddenly see her taking care of my daughter in the same place as me, while I was just trying to cope with relearning the everyday skill of grocery shopping. I tried not to show it, though, and Debra remained stoic as usual. My little one looked surprised, but untroubled.

"Deb! You caught me practising grocery shopping!"

We exchanged uncomfortable pleasantries, and then I let go of my shopping cart-walker before carefully completing a few sidesteps so I could embrace my daughter and kiss her forehead.

"Poppa Hen will be bringing you back home soon," I murmured into her soft, blond hair, trying to smother my heartbreak over my inability to do routine things for her that are second nature to most mothers.

10

Returning to Work

Shortly before being discharged from Saint-Vincent Hospital, I received a kind phone call from a human resources officer at Export Development Corporation (EDC). She proceeded to explain that their long-term disability health coverage included a rehabilitative return to the workplace, where I could come back on a part-time basis, for example. This news buoyed me; at that point, I had absolutely no idea when I would be ready to deal with returning to work, but before my stroke, my master plan had been to be a new mom working on an upwardly mobile communications career.

In my work before my stroke, I had already flown across Canada to manage the organization and local production logistics of a series of seminars for exporters; participated in advertising photo shoots; brainstormed for ad campaigns; helped set up EDC's in-house advertising agency; did media placement for the Corporation's print ads; and wrote ad copy and the odd speech.

"Oh, I really like the idea of a part-time return … at least eventually," I said hesitantly. I'd be coming back to a fast-paced, hectic environment. How would I ever be able to do it again?

"Please, take all the time you need, Cathy," she assured me. "Our rehabilitation plan lasts for two years following the date of disability. When you're ready to come in and talk to us about it some more, you can get in touch with (name withheld); she will be looking after you."

"Okay, thanks very much," I said, scribbling down the phone number dictated to me in scraggly numbers that looked like those of a four-year-old. I read them back to make sure I could read them.

Several months later, I was at the EDC office to have my chat with the nameless agent of "Inhuman" Resources. I remember hearing she had recently rebounded from a serious accident, so I was hopeful that she would be able to relate to my situation. My hopes were high for progress on getting back to work in some form, fairly soon.

But as soon as she uttered her first words after exchanging perfunctory friendly greetings, I knew I was doomed.

"Communications has undergone a major reorganization while you've been away," she began. "And unfortunately, your position has been abolished."

My mouth dropped open. "Abolished? How is that even possible?"

She shrugged. "Organizations do it all the time," she said flatly.

"And as you probably know, virtually all our other employees are involved with international financing, which requires an MBA. So, we're very sorry that the only other position we can offer you would be as an administrative assistant."

She smiled blandly, awaiting my response.

I couldn't believe what I was hearing. "But that's not … and I can't even type right now."

"Oh, you'll be surprised how much you'll be able to adapt," she said casually. "It was tough for me too, but I got through it."

Anger coursed through me. While she might indeed have a disability, it was still an ignorant, insensitive comment.

I held less against her for parroting the Corporation's neanderthal, bank-like human resources mentality (at that time), but I deeply resented her lumping me in with her own fractured perceptions of disability. She had absolutely no idea what my disabilities were; she hadn't even asked! Even if she'd had neurological issues as a result of her accident, no two brain injuries bring exactly the same symptoms or outcomes. Everyone experiences the consequences of brain trauma differently.

I had to get out of her office before I exploded, or burst into tears. I knew this was all wrong. I needed to retreat and figure things out before saying anything stupid.

"This is a lot to process," I murmured. I struggled to my feet. "I'll have to think about it for a little while."

"Of course, Cathy. Take all the time you need," she said, flashing a smile I perceived as insincere. "Thank you for coming in, and I look forward to talking with you again soon."

Yeah, I'll bet …

I already knew I would never see her again.

* * *

I made an appointment to see Dr. Clifford, and he was aghast to hear what the HR counsellor at EDC had told me.

"Cathy, I know a good lawyer. He's a friend of mine. He would gladly see you for a free consult, and from what you've told me, I think you'd have excellent grounds to take them to court, if that's what you decide to do," he said.

"That's so kind of you," I said. "I'm so confused right now. My biggest fear is that taking them to court will get me bogged down in negativity; it's so counterintuitive for keeping a progressive attitude. I still need to work through this."

He nodded soberly. "Do keep me in the loop. I'll be happy to help out any way I can."

* * *

I did meet with Dr. Clifford's lawyer friend, and I also consulted with a big law firm, now known as Nelligan Law. Both confirmed emphatically that I had grounds to sue.

Legal proceedings were for me a last resort, though, because I knew I could never go back to a place where it was evident they clearly didn't want to bother with me.

That's when I first realized that nobody is indispensable.

Export Development Corporation was a federal Schedule D Crown Corporation and operated essentially as an international export financing bank, so it wasn't required to follow the same strict employment criteria required of most federal public service departments like Transport Canada or Health Canada.

I'd always been interested in environmental responsibility, so that summer, I volunteered a couple of mornings a week at Pollution Probe, a grass-roots non-profit organization, where I conducted a survey amongst their members to identify the most critical issues they should focus on and the best approaches they could take.

It turned out that Jean-Pierre Perrier, one of my husband's childhood friends who had his own human resources consulting business, unexpectedly called me one morning.

"I have a potential lead for you," he said. "The office of the Solicitor General of Canada has a three-month opening for a part-time, entry-level human resources officer to conduct a survey for them, probably three days a week. I explained your situation to Louise Staranczak, who would be your supervisor."

"Wow! Merci, Jean-Pierre!"

"Louise is a wonderful person. I think you'll really like her."

Human resources was not my dream area to work in, but it was an appropriate rehabilitative assignment. I wasn't sure if I would ever be able to survive in a frenzied, fast-paced communications environment again, but I would be able to apply my marketing research experience, as I would be authoring a report in this assignment. It felt like a great way to see if I could ease back into handling the basic daily activities of living necessary to hold down an office job, like showering, dressing, making breakfast and commuting by car. It would also help me determine if I could last a whole day at the office without crashing or needing to lie down, and still have enough mental bandwidth to focus on the work at hand after successfully engineering the placement of my butt in the office chair.

It turned out that Louise Staranczak and I did hit it off, and Dr. Clifford wrote a touching letter of reference for me. "I know this patient very well, and I have every confidence in her," he said.

We agreed I would go to the office on Monday, Wednesday and Friday each week. On Tuesday and Thursday, I would get to "relax and rejig" at home with my little girl. (However, I will be the first to agree with many moms who say that going to work felt like a "rest" from home. At the best of times, it's a difficult balance, especially for a guilt-ridden, first-time mom saddled with life-changing disabilities that sap her self-confidence, day-in and day-out.)

When I reviewed the Solicitor General's letter of offer, I noticed that the starting salary was a tad lower than what I'd been making as a junior marketing services officer at EDC, so I mentioned this to Louise, and asked if I could receive the next increment permitted for this different occupational group, given my previously acquired experience.

"Oh yes, of course, we can certainly arrange that," Louise said.

The very next day, the phone rang. On the other end of the line was another nameless, faceless voice from Guess Who?

EDC.

"Good morning Cathy. How are you doing?"

"I'm fine," I said carefully.

"We would like to offer you your old job back. Would you be interested in coming in to discuss it with your marketing manager?"

A fiendish grin spread across my face. It was all I could do not to burst out laughing.

Louise must have called EDC to verify my previous salary. Being fluent in risk-management issues, particularly with regard to potentially litigious matters, EDC's head honchos must have woken up to an alarm from their Vice President of Human Resources and determined that since I was in the process of bailing to a more flexible government department, there was an equally high risk that I might intend to pursue legal action against them. And so by Executive Order, EDC parachuted into its risk-mitigation strategy.

But why not let them sweat a little bit, first?

"Oh! Thank you so much!" I finally chirped. "Sure, I'll come in to talk with him."

The Corporation had just moved into a shiny, brand new office tower, custom built to impress its potential foreign clientele and accommodate its growing contingent of swanky-suited export-financing soldiers. It was indeed an impressive skyscraper.

A few days later, I made my way through the cavernous glass lobby, rode up to the 13th floor, exchanged excited smiles and nods with Lynne (Normand) Hébert, one of Marketing's hardworking administrative cohorts, and knocked on the corner of my former boss's open door.

"Hey there."

"Mr. Cool" looked up at me through his aviator glasses. Underneath his tawny mustache, his smile seemed genuine. Nothing had changed.

"Hey there, Cath, come on in!" He took one last drag of his cigarette and butted it out in one of the round, brown-glassed communal ashtrays that were a fixture in every government office in those days. "So good to see you again! Have a seat. Let's talk."

"Thanks." Carefully, I placed myself in the chair facing him.

"So, how are you doing?"

"Not too bad now, compared to before," I said vaguely. "Getting better every day."

"Oh that's good, good … " He began to purposefully rearrange a few papers on his desk, signalling that our "Big Conversation" was about to start. He slowly leaned back in his high-backed chair, feigning a relaxed air.

"So," he began. "You do realize that you'll have to start at the bottom again."

"No, I won't," I said quietly and struggled to my feet. "I just came in to tell you to your face that I've found another position where the people are much more respectful, and actually give a rat's ass about their colleagues."

I wish I'd had the guts to enjoy the sight of his mouth dropping open a little longer before I marched out.

I must note that since 2002, Export Development Canada has been recognized as being among the top-100 employers in Canada. I hope that their experience with me in 1985 contributed in some small way to their becoming a more flexible, equal-opportunity employer that respects diversity.

11

From *Dogs in Canada* to Secretary of State

My three-month assignment at the office of the Solicitor General passed without fanfare. I submitted my research report and found the most difficult expectation of the job was to stand around the coffee machine making uncomfortable small talk. When it was my turn to serve myself, everyone carefully took a few steps away from me and gawked while I placed my cup on the table, clumsily poured myself half a cup of brew with my steadier left hand, then put the urn back, picked up the cup as a lefty again and carefully steered myself away from the throng. It wasn't their fault; I was still just so uncomfortable with the process of getting myself a coffee without spilling it, let alone taking a sip while standing, that I couldn't be sociable. Couldn't walk and talk at the same time …

The only thing that kept me going was that I felt happiest when I was writing. I also knew that the only way I would ever get a paying writer's job in Ottawa without a university degree would be to practise, practise, practise and submit, submit, submit until I got published, so that I could say with conviction that I was a published writer.

So when my Solicitor General term ended, I decided to stay home, take care of my little girl and write CONSTANTLY until my two-year disability pension ran out. I bought a used IBM Selectric typewriter and completed a correspondence fiction-writing course. I wrote a ridiculous novel about a brash young man who falls in love with Aileen Foster, his prudish astrologer who was 20 years his senior. She keeps pushing him away until she spots an upcoming series of nasty planetary transits in his birth chart, foretelling his imminent demise, but alas, she is too late. The young man dies in his Porsche on Highway 417 while listening to Jim Morrison belt out "Don't you love her madly."

I did get an agent from Florida, but it never got published.

Nor did any of my short stories get published, although I did receive a nod of approval from my family doctor and a bolstering note from a *Canadian Living* editor on a piece I wrote about a son and his mother in the beginning stages of Alzheimer's. It was about to go to press when something better popped up, and they had to kill it.

I did eventually get one short piece of satire published in the magazine *Dogs in Canada,* entitled "Gone to the Dogs," making fun of all the metaphorical ways the word "dog" is abused.

This gave me enough confidence to call myself a published writer on my resumé. Then, wouldn't you know it – public service employment contractor Jean-Pierre Perrier called again to let me know there was an immediate opening for a full-time writer-editor at the Department of the Secretary of State of Canada, in Ministerial Correspondence.

Perfect. I knew I could handle editing and creating short pieces in a prescribed format, so I jumped at the chance. I also knew the physical toll of working a five-day week would be devastating, but I had to believe in myself and try – and I'm so glad I did.

At Secretary of State, I met my first mentor, the late George Brimmell, and what a cheerful, iconic journalist he was! On September 11, 1961, he broke his story, "This is the Diefenbunker," in the *Toronto Telegram,* where he revealed that in the tiny town of Carp, an hour's drive from Ottawa, our federal government was building a top-secret subterranean nuclear fallout shelter. While the massive concrete structure was repeatedly officially identified as a Canadian military communications bunker, George remained skeptical. So, he hired a plane for an unauthorized fly-over with the late photographer Ted Grant, who snapped definitive proof: a massive number of toilets were about to be brought inside the structure, so George deduced it had to be something bigger, and he got the "go" to publish. He was the first to coin it the "Diefenbunker."

Apparently Prime Minister John Diefenbaker was then so incensed with this embarrassing national security leak, he demanded that George be fired from the *Telegram.* But George kept his job. There was even a PBS documentary made about his discovery, and in all the spots where George himself is interviewed, a mischievous twinkle glints in his eyes.

George also covered the assassination of President Kennedy, the first Moon landing and the Watergate scandal. He penned articles in the Canadian news magazine *Maclean's* and other leading publications, and he was a lifetime member of the Royal Ottawa Golf Club. At least once a year, he treated me to lunch there or at another restaurant close to wherever he happened to be working. He was definitely a more open and enjoyable father-figure to me than my own Dad. George was a self-made, seasoned journalist who relished the roller-coaster ride of his younger years in the news media; yet, he enjoyed every minute of his twilight years, accruing his easier, pensionable time in the federal public service.

He started me off with the easy stuff first – editing a sentence or two of a standard form-letter response – then he rapidly assigned me more and more complex tasks, to the point where I essentially wrote the entire letter.

"You've got quite the knack," he said jovially. "How would you like to try writing an article for the department's newsletter on the progress of negotiations for new contracts with our various occupational groups? I sure don't want to do it!"

After that assignment, I was given the opportunity to write my first investigative piece, which I did largely on my own, with gentle guidance from George. When it was published, I was delighted to find a photocopy of it waiting for me on my desk, scrolled with the words "Good work, Cathy! D. Christensen," from our branch's Director General. I was humbled, as this was the first personal contact from an executive who terrified me. As a matter of fact, all executives terrified me. One of my biggest psychological impairments was that I often felt like an imposter without a university degree.

* * *

Earlier in my career, when I had worked in advertising at EDC, one of the creative pursuits I found most satisfying was synthesizing big-picture concepts into awesome one-liners such as slogans, head-lines and titles.

One of my greatest thrills at Secretary of State came when I was asked to participate in a brainstorming session to come up with the best slogan to promote a new annual event that is now known as International Day for Persons with Disabilities, on December 3. This was the kind of exercise I loved!

For over an hour, I listened to six earnest, well-meaning individuals batting big ideas back and forth, peppered with musings as to whether the word "disability" should be included, while contemplating that the idea of "accessibility for all" had to be paramount, and yada yada yada …

After a protracted pause, indicating a temporary exhaustion of good intentions, I gathered the courage to pipe up.

"How about we say something like 'Independence: That's Living!'"

They all stared at me, the burden gradually lifting from their faces.

"That sounds perfect!" group leader Sandra Souchotte gushed.

The others dared to smile harder and nod more quickly.

On another occasion, George was particularly delighted with a piece I wrote on how royal visits were organized at Secretary of State, after I interviewed the director responsible for the ins and outs of the plethora of protocols.

"You should send this out to newspaper editors, especially in cities who've received royal visits," he suggested, and so I did. There was no pick-up, but to my surprise, I received a couple of "kill fees" from dailies in western Canada. In other words, I wouldn't get a byline, but they were rewarding me as a legitimate source for their own writers.

(Ironically, the late Prime Minister Brian Mulroney had named no one other than Lucien Bouchard as the Secretary of State while I was working there. Less than two years later, Monsieur Bouchard formed le Bloc Québécois, served as leader of the Official Opposition, and then later became Premier of Quebec. Hardly a fan of the monarchy, I would think.)

I absolutely loved my time working at Secretary of State, but there inevitably came a point where I could no longer fulfil the requirement to be physically present from Monday to Friday. I asked Director Marion Brown if there was any chance I could scale down to four days a week. (This was eons before the "flexible work week" became a viable option, let alone morphing into the new home office normality spawned from the COVID-19 pandemic as an economic and life-saving necessity that forced even the most conventional workplaces to think outside the box.)

"Unfortunately, we're just not set up for that," Marion said kindly, "But we'd certainly hire you for all sorts of projects on contract as a freelancer. That way, you could work at home and just come in to deliver your stuff or to interview someone."

It was a wonderful idea! Our little girl was thriving in kindergarten, and she could stay with our next-door neighbour for a short time on those random days when I knew I could not make it back in time to meet her school bus.

I accepted Marion's offer without hesitation. I knew they liked me and would continue to keep me busy enough to do what I loved, at home. I felt so proud to be my own boss for a couple of years.

I continued to write articles for the Secretary of State newsletter and the odd speech, and then other federal departments began to call, particularly the Medical Research Council, with communications headed by Denis St-Jean.

Denis, a former Secretary of State executive, also continued to show a long-term supportive interest in me. He faithfully sent me Christmas cards for many years, even after vaulting up the corporate ladder to manage communications for the Ottawa Hospital. (From there, he offered me a position as a part-time communicator for the Royal Ottawa Rehabilitation Centre. However, this happened after my second, more serious stroke, so I turned it down, thinking at that point that I would never work again.)

Another sweet freelancing stint was an assignment to clear a backlog of Ministerial correspondence in the Office of Joe Clark, who at that time was responsible for the Canadian International

Development Agency. I could work my own hours, but I had to be physically present, since the work environment was classified as "secret." My glass-walled office overlooked the majestic Ottawa River from Place du Portage, in Gatineau, Quebec, and it was just a quick jaunt across the Macdonald-Cartier Bridge to the Rockcliffe Parkway, and back to the beautiful home we had just purchased in a wooded neighbourhood in Orléans. I revelled in the experience as I drove my car back and forth to the office, up, around and down that twisty cliff – albeit in daylight – thinking how I had come such a long way since the night its streetlights made me dizzy and nauseous when I came back home for the first time from Saint-Vincent hospital, nearly six years ago. Life was good!

Round II

12

July 31, 1990: Not Again!

Six years after my first stroke, to look at me, you would see no visible clues I'd had one. My stride gave no hint of an altered gait, and my smile at that time looked completely straight. As long as I remembered to keep a sharp eye on my right hand, it was a willing and fairly capable supporter of my now more-dominant left hand, with which I now took a pen to write without even thinking. I even ventured out for the occasional short bike ride around the block, with my right foot inserted into a metal clamp on the pedal so it wouldn't fly off. (Those rides didn't last long, though; I just couldn't balance enough to feel safe.)

In March 1987, my daughter (now 3 ½ years old) and I enjoyed our first solo getaway to Vancouver. We spent some precious time with my parents and she got to meet her great-grandfather David Driedger and his lovely second wife, Edith.

We resumed family camping trips every summer throughout Eastern Canada and the Maritimes, and had crazy fun camping at Charleston Lake, Ontario, and Oka, Quebec, with our daughter's caregiver, Debra Laxton, her husband Doug, and their three kids. Whenever the weather and time allowed, the Allards would venture out for many a picnic all over the Ottawa-Gatineau area, and we always went apple picking (especially for the hot, homemade mini-doughnuts that came along with the activity) in the fall.

I loved working as a freelance writer. As long as I stuck to my "one big thing a day" mantra and paced myself accordingly – by taking a break before I got tired – my energy levels had markedly improved. Much easier said than done, though. If there was a sustained combination of too many late nights and too much excitement, or if I tried to squeeze too many activities into one day or got too much sunshine, I would invariably end up unloading the contents of my stomach with a massive two-day migraine. When this happened, I was forced to lie down behind closed doors in a dark, quiet bedroom, until I could keep down enough sips of water to risk taking the medications that allowed me to feel remotely functional again.

But being alive, loving my family, working again and being able to participate, both with them and independently, as well as doing basic things that one might not even consider to be a challenge – like riding in a car or driving, let alone with a left-foot gas pedal – felt glorious. For the most part, I was back to my pre-stroke self, and my struggles were largely memories relegated to the distant past.

It turned out to be the classic calm before the storm.

⋆ ⋆ ⋆

It was the summer between Grade 1 and Grade 2 for our daughter. She and her Poppa Hen were enjoying an after-dinner dip at the Gloucester wave pool, while I was in our upstairs office working on a brochure for the Canadian International Development Agency. I was attempting this task in the midst of a raging migraine headache.

It was a doozy. As I stared at my computer screen, I was taunted by intense, random patterns of crazy zigzags, making reading impossible. I lowered my head, closed my eyes, massaged the bridge of my nose, and cursed. Further work on the brochure copy was a no-go. I knew I was headed for another one of those three-day, barf-fest clusterfucks, where no light, sound, food or water could be tolerated.

Again, "stupid me" had overdone it the day before, insisting that I was just fine trimming our backyard cedar hedges with a hard-to-handle chainsaw, while perched precariously on a stepladder under the broiling sun, with a humidex of 33 degrees Celsius.

Still, this nausea jolted me with alarming intensity. I sprang up and hurried down the hallway, the vomit erupting in convulsions the moment I made it to the toilet.

Migraine barfing was part of my family heritage, but this was all wrong. This was not my usual migraine experience – something different was occurring. Panic set in.

I already knew it was another stroke.

Have to get to the phone …

Call 911 …

I staggered back to the office, barely grabbed the receiver, and collapsed.

I have no idea how much time passed before the two loves of my life returned home to find their worlds shattered. Again. In my semi-conscious, panicked, jumbled mind, random thoughts darted around me …

Just hang in there … you can't move, but you MUST be okay … have to be … they'll be home soon … they'll find you, and then everything'll be okay … Ohhhh … I am so fucked up again … but must be strong … must protect my little girl … must explain it to her … she's so smart … it's what happened last time … you were just a baby … only a stroke … and I came back … must make her understand … I am not dead … still here … I will never abandon her …

I heard the key turn in the front door, and they pranced inside, all happy and unsuspecting.

I managed to call out her name. "Ccommmme … ere … "

I saw only the top of her blonde head bouncing up the stairs. When she discovered me contorted on the floor, I heard her horrified cries, all hell broke loose, and everything faded to black …

* * *

A few years afterwards, I learned my daughter felt as if my calling out to her had been a mean trick, that I had lured her upstairs on false pretences. That was the last thing I'd meant to do, but that's how a stroke can screw up your thinking. Deep down, I was probably terrified of dying without seeing her again, while clinging to that fleeting glimpse of the top of her head.

* * *

The next memory came two days later, back in the neuro ward at the General Hospital. Jean-Pierre implored me to let him help me out of bed and walk with me to use the toilet. I was unwilling at first; I just wanted to use the bedpan, but he kept on insisting. So finally, I acquiesced.

When I tried to stand, I could not get my right foot to rest flat on the floor. The ankle, all twisted, forced the foot to land on its outer edge, making every step excruciatingly painful, even with JP practically carrying me.

"Try to straighten out your foot," he coaxed.

"C-c- anti … mmabba … maba … hummm … humba … "

I knew I was babbling gibberish. Worse, I had no idea what I was trying to say. Jean-Pierre looked horrified, as if I had just shot him in the chest.

Oh, dear God … I'm aphasic … can't speak properly … and I have no control of my right ankle, or my foot. They're paralyzed.

We struggled silently the rest of the way to the toilet, and he helped me drop my drawers and do my business.

"Let's get you back into bed," he said tonelessly, near tears.

* * *

The CAT scan confirmed our fears – it was another cerebrovascular accident – another stroke.

Soon after, I was surprised to get a one-minute visit in the hospital from my family doctor.

"We need to try to find out WHY it happened," he said. It took everything I had to hide my rage. I had already decided to change family doctors because I felt this one had let me down.

At least six months before the second stroke, his nurse had noted on more than one occasion that my blood pressure was elevated after I climbed the stairs to his office. However, no hypertension meds were ever prescribed.

In all fairness though, this doctor had helped me a great deal after my first stroke. He prescribed me a small dose of amitriptyline to take at bedtime, which did a wonderful job of calming the burning sensations on my right side so that I could sleep through the night. On the rare occasions when I missed a dose, I could never fall asleep, and before dawn, I'd know that the coming day was doomed to hellfire. He gave me great, objective counselling about getting my life back together, and he even willingly reviewed my short story on Alzheimer's for accuracy before *Canadian Living* killed it at the last-minute.

He also prescribed me Imitrex injections for my debilitating migraine headaches (a good 15 years before Ottawa Hospital's Stroke Prevention Clinic told me to stop taking it, citing research determining that the drug increased the risk of stroke).

He was kind and supportive, but I was disappointed that nothing had been done to deal with my high blood pressure. Could the hypertension have contributed to this second stroke?

The team at the Ottawa Hospital wanted to discover the WHY, but I didn't co-operate with all their investigative plans.

My doctors there wanted to do another neurological angiogram, but I flatly refused. I would not submit to another life-threatening procedure. To my mind, it was a stroke, plain and simple, either from a blood clot or a severe migraine.

Medical research journals indicate that while migrainous blood clots causing strokes are rare – and their causes are not fully understood – they occur most often in people who have regular migraines with aura. Additionally, women under the age of 45 appear to be at a greater risk, particularly those who have taken oral contraceptives and smoked.

Bottom line: there were no magicians around anywhere to reverse it.

Every morning, the residents would arrive, poke around my foot, and politely command me to try to move it. But their requests held none of the magic of Dr. Mallya. Nothing was improving.

Fortunately, my muddled brain never mixed up spoken or written words again after that early encounter with JP. I cannot even begin to express how grateful I am for that.

Again, I was transferred to Saint-Vincent Hospital for rehabilitation. I was not surprised by this. Somehow, my right foot had been twisted sideways, with the big toe pointing upwards in the opposite direction, and I couldn't put any weight on it without the whole leg seizing up from the stabbing pain coming from the side of the foot that made contact with the ground. All I knew was that I had to try to get better, and Saint-Vincent's was the best place for that.

I did not sit in the front seat with the ambulance driver this time.

However, like the last time, the first day did not get off to a good start. In fact, I was almost sent back to the General that night, after I projectile-vomited all over the poor nurse who was bathing me. They must have checked my file to discover that for me, this was business as usual.

The entire healthcare team was new, except for Head Nurse Sandi Millar. My physiatrist was a soft-spoken, very kind man, but he always appeared to be stressed out and uncomfortable.

At the first get-to-know-your-treatment-team visit, I declined psychological and social work sessions. Been there, done that. I knew exactly what I would be facing. Especially after Sandi Millar passed me a little post-it note of encouragement from my former psychologist, Céline Paris, who just happened to be visiting Saint-Vincent's the day before I was readmitted. That was enough for me to know who was in my corner.

That first night on ward 1D, I couldn't sleep. After everyone had gone to bed, I got myself into my wheelchair. I needed to figure out how to push myself around. My plan was to make it to the end of the hall and back; hopefully by then, I would be more than ready to pass out.

With hemiparesis, or one weakened side, it can be exceedingly difficult to propel your wheelchair in a straight line. The stronger arm tends to turn the chair in circles because the weaker arm has less force. I ended up pushing myself as hard as I could with my left arm, and then trying to steer back on course with weaker, multiple pushes from the right. Good thing the dark hallway was empty.

I reached the end of the hall and came to rest in front of a noticeboard outside the physiotherapy gallery. I pretended to read, in case anyone was watching, but I could not suppress my sobs of despair. I was terrified that I would spend the rest of my life in a wheelchair.

13

Leg Brace and Botox

After a few weeks, I had started taking a few crooked steps in physiotherapy, but every step of my right foot landed with a brutally painful thump on its outer periphery. Still, being up and out of the wheelchair for short periods gave me active hope that one day I wouldn't need to rely on it. It was still early, and with hard work and lots of therapy, maybe I could rise above this, just like last time …

Still, it was a huge blow when my physiatrist made a sombre announcement at the Friday team meeting. He appeared particu larly ill at ease.

"Cathy, you will need to wear a brace on your leg to ensure your stability when walking," he said.

My mouth dropped open in alarm. I wasn't expecting such a grave prognosis so soon. I thought I was making significant progress and was devastated to suddenly understand that wearing a brace would be a necessary and non-negotiable part of my rehabilitation.

"We will be sending you to a chiropodist (foot specialist) next week," he continued, with caring eyes. "He will first take a cast of your leg to make the brace. It should be ready soon after you are discharged, and you will continue to come here for outpatient physiotherapy."

I nodded, dejected. I felt crippled, inside and out.

* * *

Eventually, I would find the pain from wearing the hard, plastic one-piece ankle-foot orthosis (AFO), fastened with Velcro, was more debilitating than the stroke itself. The pain of every step tortured my psyche and completely exhausted any enjoyment of life. It was not designed to straighten my twisted foot; it was only meant to keep the ankle stable enough for me to walk. With every step, my foot's outer edge slammed against the unforgiving plastic, shooting long, agonizing electric shocks up my calf. This made the foot spasm and curl up even more in its instinctive reaction to protect itself. And the more the foot was in fight-or-flight mode, the more the big toe raised itself high in the air like an objecting toddler whose tantrums were impossible to quell.

When the chiropodist first brought out my new AFO, disappointment tore through me. The plastic brace lacked a hinge (or articulation, as it's called) at the ankle to allow for freer isolated movement of the leg, when bending the knees or when seated to put on shoes, for example. I had seen others wearing an articulated AFO and expected I would be offered something similar, but given my frozen ankle, I figured there must have been a valid medical reason why an ankle hinge was not deemed suitable for me.

Every task of daily living became exhausting.

Finding a comfortable shoe or boot was impossible; the priority was rapidly downgraded to being able to insert the braced foot with the elevated angry big toe into any shoe and satisfactorily fastening it on my own.

Independence – That's Living became the first mantra I began to tell myself every day. Hmmm, wonder where that came from … I fell into a deep depression.

I gained 40 pounds.

At 33, I often felt like my life was over.

I was fortunate enough to find a wonderful new family doctor, though. Her name was Louise Linney, and she collaborated with me for more than 20 years to carve out my bumpy path to regaining the confidence to believe in myself again and heal myself. My daughter's first caregiver, Debra Laxton, told me about her.

"Sometimes she can be abrupt, but I really like her," Debra said.

I could be abrupt sometimes too, so Louise and I got along just fine.

The first thing she did was take my blood pressure. She frowned.

"For someone with your history, this is not good," she told me. "I want you to come in for another blood pressure test next week, and the week after that, and if your readings are the same, I'm putting you on medication for hypertension. We need to reduce the risk as much as possible of you having another stroke."

That's exactly what I wanted too.

About a year later, Louise agreed to refer me to the Royal Ottawa Rehabilitation Centre's Prosthetics and Orthotics Department to fashion me an articulated brace. At last, I was being given an opportunity to move on from the stiff and painful brace that had been my burden.

Nathalie Anglehart was the amazingly talented prosthetics and orthotics artist assigned to me, and she became my superstar. The bottom of the new hinged AFO cradled my foot more like a glove, and after a couple of adjustment visits, the finished product provided more room to allow the toes to lie more placidly, helping to relax the ever-pushing-upwards big toe. The added hinge also allowed my leg to move in a more natural heel-to-toe sequence when walking. And best of all, the pain was cut in half.

Nathalie also referred me to the Rehab Centre's foot-care clinic to keep my toenails properly clipped every six weeks. It wasn't a pedicure, but it was covered by the Ontario Health Insurance Plan (OHIP), and I developed a fun routine of parking far away and walking to the clinic, rain or shine.

The foot clinic became my Safe Haven. I trusted their expertise completely.

At one of these foot-care visits, maybe a year later, manager Ruth Thompson agreed with my observation that the nail bed of my big right toe was shifting sideways, making the nail push into the skin. Even regular nail trimming would not stop the ever-increasing pressure and pain.

"I'm going to get my orthotics colleague Graham Curryer to come over and have a look," she decided. "He has a lot of surgical experience with either total or partial nail avulsion, and he'll know exactly how to handle this."

She scurried across the hall to Orthotics to snatch Graham away from another patient for a quick consult on the best way to calm my uncooperative, angry big toe. After only a few minutes, they strode back into my lab room together.

"Hi Cathy, I'm Graham. So nice to meet you!"

His friendly, intelligent smile was infectious, and his bouncing, positive energy made him instantly likeable. He cheerfully sized up my toe in about two seconds.

"Oh sure, I can do the avulsion surgery here; I'll just remove this inside part of your toenail here," he explained, pointing. "We just wrap a thick elastic band around the bottom of your toe here, freeze it with local anesthetic, permanently remove the offending area, and bingo, you'll be good to go. And no pain, except for the injection jab. Sound good?"

Little did I know how profoundly Graham's treatments, innovative ideas and recommendations would improve my life in the years to come. A couple of weeks later, in the spring of 1997, Graham completed his handiwork and removed the elastic band from my big toe with a flourish.

"Voilà, Madame!"

"Thank you. Didn't hurt a bit, just like you said."

"That's good!" He continued to peer at my foot, then looked over at my articulated brace leaning against the wall. "How are you doing with that thing?"

I grimaced. "It gets me around much better with much less

pain, but it still hurts like hell."

He nodded, deliberating, and his eyes lit up as he decided to share his revelation. "I just learned about something you might benefit from. It's still quite controversial, but I think you should go see your physiatrist and ask him to refer you for a consult."

I was intrigued. "What is it?"

"You're not going to believe this." He wore a devilish grin. "It's Botox injections. In your ankle."

Botox is made from the toxin that can lead to botulism – the toxin that can naturally occur when certain foods, particularly seafood, start to decompose, or go bad. If ingested, its poison can kill you.

My eyes widened. "Really?"

He nodded, brimming with excitement. "You know how people get it to remove wrinkles on their face? Well, it works because the Botox temporarily paralyzes or relaxes the tightened muscles that are causing the skin to bunch up and wrinkle. And from that, it's recently been scientifically proven that Botox injections can actually help reduce spasticity. Like what you have in your foot."

"Ah, I see … so my foot would relax more in the brace, and it wouldn't hurt so much."

"Yes. Exactly. We're even using it here at the Rehab Centre for children with muscular dystrophy, and I just heard that Dr. Stys, a neurologist at the Civic Hospital, has reported some success with stroke patients."

"Wow! I'll go see my physiatrist right away, then. Thank you so much!"

He raised a hand in caution. "You must be aware though; there are a lot of 'cons.' It may not work for you, and the effects are not permanent; so it would have to be done on a regular basis. Each dose is extremely expensive, and it's not covered by OHIP."

"I don't care. I have to try it."

He seemed happy to find me so enthusiastic. "Also, keep in mind that after repeated injections, its effectiveness gradually reduces," he cautioned. "And there may be a lot of doctors who will be against it right now because it's so new, and there isn't a lot of documentation out there. They might not even know about it."

"Yeah, but if you guys here know and Neurology at the Civic's doing it, that's promising."

"Just keep my cautions in mind," he repeated. "I'm really glad you're going to look into it, though. I think you'd be an excellent candidate."

* * *

It turns out Graham was right about everything.

My physical medicine and rehabilitation specialist (physiatrist) at Saint-Vincent Hospital flatly refused to refer me to the Civic Hospital's neurologist, Dr. Stys, for a Botox injection.

"Oh no, no, no," he muttered, lowering his eyes and shaking his head back and forth repeatedly, as if to expel the shock of such a ridiculous request and making it crystal clear that he could not be swayed. "I'm sorry, but I cannot recommend that. It's still experimental, I have no idea what it might do to you, and it's exorbitantly expensive."

Even with Graham's warning, I was still surprised by the

intensity of my physiatrist's dismissive response and his apparent unwillingness to consider discussing what I had learned. What I do know is that this kind man had the best intentions to protect me.

I didn't waste time, though. I discussed the big Botox affair with my family doctor, Louise Linney, and she was delighted to refer me to Dr. Stys.

* * *

Neurologist Dr. Christine De Meulemeester, an associate of Dr. Stys at the time, first assessed my intake form and then came to check me out and get to know me and my issues. Then, after she left to debrief Dr. Stys, he came in to chat. I remember he seemed fascinated when I described my reduced awareness of my body parts combined with hypersensitivity to pain, heat and cold.

"I think you could benefit quite a lot from this treatment," he said. "It's not cheap though."

"I don't care what it costs," I said, even though we were now a one-income family with our line of credit spiralling out of control, along with the grim prospect that I would likely never work ever again. The way I saw it at the time: I couldn't risk returning to the workplace. I'd never survive a third stroke. But money didn't matter; I needed to continue my recovery efforts with less relentless pain; then my brain would have more bandwidth to think past endurance and physical issues. And then I could devote more of my energies to being more present and actively enjoying a happier day-to-day life with my family.

"Each injection dose costs about $250 and lasts a minimum of three months, but it can last longer, even up to six months; it just depends on the individual," Dr. Stys explained. "The idea is to wait as long as you can between each injection; that way, the treatment itself will last longer."

"Sounds good. So what's next?"

"I'll write you a prescription now, and you can take it downstairs to the hospital pharmacy. You should call them as soon as the date of your appointment is confirmed. Then, on the day of your injection, about an hour before, you pick up the vials from the pharmacy and bring them to us; they'll give you a freezer pack to keep them cold."

"Okay, that sounds great."

He scribbled out the prescription. "It'll be Dr. Barclay who will be giving you the injections. She is very good at this and has seen some excellent results. She will probably inject in two or maybe even three different spots on your ankle the first time, and we'll see how you respond."

He passed me the prescription with a light smile. "I should warn you that the needles are large and quite long, and will be inserted quite deeply, so the injections themselves can be quite painful."

I grinned. "Like Dr. Jekyll and Mr. Hyde?"

"Well, it'll hurt, but you won't end up like Mr. Hyde," he joked. We were comparing the giant experimental needle filled with the "poison" of Botox to the horror story written by Robert Louis Stevenson in 1883, where Dr. Jekyll turns into a raging monster "Mr. Hyde" after he takes his own experimental serum.

Dr. Stys got up from his chair and shook my hand. "It was very nice meeting you, Cathy. I wish you the best."

* * *

It was a good thing Dr. Stys didn't ask me if I was afraid of needles. I really wasn't. I'd already weathered a spinal tap at Saint-Vincent Hospital to rule out multiple sclerosis, once and for all. I had to lie down for eight hours afterwards, to allow enough time for the fluid withdrawn from the base of the spine to flow back up and through the brain, so I could avoid a massive headache. However, I must admit that when I saw the size of the monster needle the cheerful Dr. Barclay was about to stick me with, a few pricks of fear shot through me.

"It usually takes a couple of days before you'll notice any changes," she said. "Are you ready?"

"Yup." I steeled myself to remain still.

"Okay now, take a slow, deep breath … "

Wickedly sharp, thick, burning metal pierced deeper and deeper into the flesh of my ankle relentlessly, making me shudder.

Oh my God is this ever going to stop … are they lying to me? Is my foot being amputated? I willed myself to keep holding my breath, hoping I would have enough lung capacity.

Then she slowly withdrew the needle, and the violation ceased. I let go a giant woosh, and she smiled at me.

"That went really well," she said. "Pretty intense though, wasn't it?"

I nodded.

"Well, good news. That one was the worst. The next two will be a lot easier."

* * *

The transformation was nothing short of miraculous.

The Botox reduced my paralyzed foot's spasticity so much that it rested almost flat on the floor, as opposed to teetering on its outer edge. And since there was less resistance in the brace, the constant slamming motion when I was walking almost disappeared, and so did the pain. Moreover, my stamina increased. I could walk longer and farther, and enjoy every day more and more.

And I could do more. I could think more. I yearned to be more active.

I felt reborn.

14

Addicted to Aquafit

Since the second stroke, JP, our daughter and I had been to the wave pool a couple of times for a family "aqua romp." I have always loved the water, even though I'd been a mediocre swimmer at best. But now, I couldn't float steadily enough to swim properly; my heavier, more dominant left side always started to sink before the right side, and my weaker right arm couldn't provide the same force to keep my body balanced. The only thing I could sustain for more than a few seconds was to float on my back. Don't get me wrong; the water felt great, but it exhausted me. Thankfully, my little sweetie was so autonomous and disciplined in the changeroom after all the fun, but it broke my heart. She was so mature for her young age, such a grown-up soul.

These family outings at the wave pool led me to recall the suggestion a physiotherapist had made to me after the first stroke six years earlier, that I should consider trying an aquafit class to help decrease pain and improve mobility. So I started to do some research on the environment that might work best for me. To my delight, I discovered that there was a "light" aquafit class offered at the Orléans Recreation Centre, just down the hill from our house. The best part was the warm therapy pool. It accommodated only one class at a time, with gloriously warm, soothing, chest-high water. Its wide, textured, slip-proof stairs with handlebars on both sides made the descent almost as easy as a flight of stairs at home. Enjoying a 45-minute bath to fun music with a little dancing thrown in would be such a treat!

Wearing laced-up aqua shoes with the heaviest treads I could find and gripping the handle of the trusty cane I used for "rough terrain," which included a slippery-when-wet surface, I took a deep breath, summoned all my courage and hobbled out onto the pool deck.

I gawked at all the smiling older women chatting on the benches and floating languidly on noodles in the pool, waiting for the class to start. *Looks like I'm the youngest … again …*

Before I figured out how to safely make my way into the water, a pair of smiling ladies approached and welcomed me. Gail McDermid and Pat Kelly instantly made me feel like I belonged. We became a cherished "aqua-trio" for 12 more years, and lifelong friends.

Pat and Gail were two of the original participants of the new light aquafit program when it was first introduced, and they loyally attended every Tuesday and Thursday – staving off continued threats to cancel the program due to low attendance. This was a good decade before exercising in the water became the sexy and best no-impact way for aerobics addicts, seniors and others with physical issues to have fun dancing in the water.

Gail, a former nurse, was smart, simple and no-nonsense, and she had a warped sense of humour like me. She thoroughly enjoyed her affectionate reputation as a "slacker." Near the end of the 45-minute class, Gail could nearly always be found floating languidly on a brightly coloured foam noodle, with a smug grin on her face – long before jovial group leader Mark Shwartz announced to the roughly six to eight women who were still working hard in the pool that it was cool-down time.

Pat was one of the dearest, most caring women I have ever known; she was unconditionally devoted to her family, often at her own expense. Sadly, during the pandemic, she lived with pancreatic cancer for two years, and before passing away, she spent every possible moment with her husband Ted, daughter Lisa and her three granddaughters, the lights of her life.

Gail and Pat first met when their daughters attended elementary school together.

It wasn't long before I was joining Pat and Gail at a nearby Harvey's restaurant for coffee and sometimes even breakfast before the 10 a.m. start time. Then, after class, most of the ladies would meet up at Country Style Donuts for some more caffeine, more chatting and perhaps a sweet reward to sabotage our "sustained" efforts. Meanwhile, Pat, Gail and I secretly plotted where we would go, just the three of us, for our "A-Team" lunch, if we hadn't already figured that out in the pool. There were always one or two women whom we did NOT want to dine with.

I know, so catty …

We all loved Mark Schwartz, our tall, sweetly hilarious lifeguard and therapy-pool leader. His long, curly brown locks flowed past his shoulders, framing his friendly face. He reminded me of saxophonist Kenny G. He always made us laugh and forget our troubles.

Mark stayed with our group for a few years. I think he took a tad longer to finish university because he was having so much fun – especially with his risky obsession with rock climbing – but eventually, he moved on from his limping, tittering ladies with bad hips, hearts and head injuries. Then, Elaine Rhodenizer, of similar age to most of us, became our new leader.

Elaine's waterproof, articulated knee brace was the only outward sign of her debilitating chronic physical issues. With a Bachelor's in Kinesiology, she worked at the YM-YWCA in her younger years and was an avid skier until she smashed up one of her legs in a horrific accident on the slopes. So for Elaine, teaching aquafit in the water was her own essential "heal-thyself" therapy. She taught me a great deal about how to remain resolved during those times when everything hurts so much you just want to go to sleep and never wake up.

Dear Elaine rallied us to work as hard as we could, and she'd demonstrate easier or more appropriate options for those with hip replacements, or whatever else ailed us. She too had a great sense of humour, but she was more insistent about us making the most of our time in the water. Sometimes when Elaine was having a bad day, or if Gail was overdoing her noodle chatter, Elaine would frostily advise us to ease off the chit-chat until the cool-down period at the end of the class.

To this day, Elaine remains a dear friend. She once told me that of all the aquafit participants she has led over the years, I was the one who had shown the most improvement. Nowadays, we don't get to see each other as often as we'd like, but whenever I think of her, I am honoured to be reminded of how important it is to keep working on the skills you possess and to find ways to keep it fun.

15

Enjoying Our Kitchen

I also started to enjoy playing in the kitchen again, preparing delicious, healthy meals for our little family – largely thanks to the late aquafit participant Denise Poulin, also taken from us too soon by cancer. Denise told me about *Canadian Living* nutrition editor and cookbook author Anne Lindsay and encouraged me to get a copy of her book, *Lighthearted Everyday Cooking,* produced in partnership with the Heart and Stroke Foundation. Anne Lindsay's commitment to easy, delicious and nutritious recipes was a perfect fit for me, and for about five years, I spent most weekday afternoons preparing her easy recipes to delight my tiny family with delicious dishes.

Chicken stew with dumplings; Indonesian fried rice; salmon loaf with dill; lamb, spinach and feta in pita pockets; make-ahead turkey divan; black bean quesadillas … Mmm Mmm!

I still make recipes in lots of little steps and take frequent breaks. I often sit down to chop up a mess of onions or zest a lemon. Or I find a smaller cup to slowly transfer hot liquids to another vessel, since my numb hand is not very good at hanging onto a huge, heavy bowl while simultaneously manoeuvering it to aim somewhere else specific – particularly if the liquid is hot or the emptying requires grasping a wooden spoon or spatula. From time to time, you have to adopt those Cirque du Soleil moves. There can be arguing too, when Poppa Hen wants to "help me do something" I know I can do on my own. (I usually let him take over when it involves taking something hot and heavy out of the oven.) When he sees me working in the kitchen, he automatically worries that I am struggling, but I'm just doing it my own way.

I think it might be fair to say that my enthusiastic adventures in the kitchen played a small role in influencing my hubby and daughter to become the skilled chefs and good food addicts they are today.

When our daughter was 11, she made a braided challah loaf. All by herself.

On weekends, she moved into true restaurant mode. After she'd whipped up dinner for three, she pushed JP and me out the front door and ordered us to wait for our appointed reservation time before ringing the doorbell.

We rang, and our "maître d" promptly opened the door and bowed to us, a dish towel carefully draped at her wrist.

"Good evening," she said officiously. "Would you have a reservation?"

"Yes, Jean Blanc-le-Blanc, party of two, for 7 p.m."

She checked her list. "Ah, yes. Excellent." She offered us two small cards, both immaculately titled "Table d'hôte," listing all the courses, house wine and other beverages on offer that evening. "Please, follow me. I will bring you to your table."

Linens, placemats, cutlery and drinking vessels for three were all precisely arranged. We were also assured that our "maître d" had taste-tested "un soupçon" of each dish before plating to ensure it was palate-worthy for her customers.

The food was exquisite.

She has since matured into a certifiable foodie. For more than 15 years, she has been a founding member of a group called "the Four Fs" (Fabulous Foodie Femmes & Friends), composed of dear friends she made when she started her public service career in Ottawa.

Excluding their envious partners, the Four Fs get together several times a year at one of the member's homes, where they meticulously cook, drink, consume and celebrate an outrageously-themed evening, chosen by the host. Uber brings everyone home safely.

16

Making Progress, One Slow
Step at a Time

After the Botox injections relieved much of the pain of my twisted foot in the leg brace, and my stamina increased, my self-confidence grew. I felt more inspired to more regularly drive to our local grocery store and buy our family's weekly groceries. With higher energy levels, I was also able to stretch myself when it came to the daily activities of my own physical care; I moved beyond yanking on a sweatsuit to experimenting with fastening blue jeans, with their cold metal zippers and waist buttons, and to wearing long-sleeved shirts with cuffs – which posed their own unique challenges.

The cuffs needed to be loose enough for me to button up the left one before I put on the shirt, since my right fingers were too clumsy to complete the task. The material had to feel good on my right side, too. Often, I would be sweltering on my left side, while stinging and freezing on my right. This led me to further master the "hemiparesis (neurological impairment affecting one side of the body)-look cardigan-scarf" sweater – with my right arm in its sleeve, and the left swung around my neck and over my right shoulder – and ta-da … I felt stylish and comfy, and better prepared to take on the world.

But despite my progress, I still couldn't see myself ever being able to cope in a 9-to-5 environment. That was simply impossible right now, even though we were now without my freelance writing income, and our line of credit kept increasing every month.

This period my daughter and I shared together one-on-one was tender and for the most part, calm, although I felt as if there was an emotional wall between us – a lot of unarticulated frustrations on both our parts, possibly because I couldn't just go to cuddle her spontaneously or pull her away from danger. Like the time she stood up on her tiptoes, gleefully reaching over the kitchen counter to grab hold of the big can of pretty peaches I was trying to open, and then, as the can slipped off the counter and smashed her big toenail into a bloody mess, her horrified screams of agony punctured my heart. She was so willful sometimes, and I felt so woefully incompetent.

Something else I'm not proud of: sometimes, after a sinfully tasty lunch of boxed macaroni and cheese, with a giant tablespoon of extra bottled cheese sauce and cut up hot dogs thrown into the sauce, along with huge globs of ketchup on the side, we would descend to the basement to have our afternoon rest in front of *Days of our Lives.* Ah, the romances of Beautiful Bo and Sexy Hope; the Glamorous Marlena teasing her Steadfast Roman, and Sweet Kayla and her Blond Swashbuckler Patch filled an hour of pleasant escape from our own realities. Most of the time, my little darling sat with me, engrossed, especially whenever Patch was on. But she'd often loosen herself from my side and march over to her little wooden desk with two chairs to draw, colour or play with her beloved red Dictée Magique, a talking French spelling machine. Its robotic male voice with a clipped Parisian accent emanating from its red plastic speaker was an oddly comforting sound throughout our house.

Bonjour. Épeler "fromage." (Good day. Spell "cheese.")

Her tiny fingers replied rapidly on the keypad, displaying her chosen letters on the small, lined screen.

Bonne réponse (right answer), replied the French judge and moderator. *Maintenant, épeler "moitié."* (Now, spell "half.") Click clickety click …

Ce n'est pas une bonne réponse. Essayez encore. (That is not the right answer. Try again.) She entered her second of three tries.

Bonne réponse.

Tu a gagné. (You won!)

She always found a constructive way to amuse herself. But deep down, I loathed myself.

I was behaving exactly like my languishing, invalid mother had done with me. She had been addicted to *The Edge of Night*, and there wasn't much else for me to do in my sparse environment but join her in front of the TV to watch the drama unfold. I remember vowing to myself that if I ever had kids, I would never subject them to watching soap operas.

Yet here I was, doing exactly the same thing to my own daughter. I hated myself for that, although it did bring me more understanding of what my Mom had felt.

Once I realized how easy it is to repeat what you learn, I vowed, perhaps out of flawed logic, that if I ever found a way to make it back to work, I would never watch another soap opera again.

Hah! Why are you even THINKING about going back to work? Because you're such an inadequate mother? You've never been naturally maternal … you were always a Type A achiever; you always wanted to show your Mom that you would never be satisfied living your life as a victim. And what a competent, strong, independent professional you were, despite the challenges you faced to reach that point …

There were so many more happy playtimes with ma petite amour, though. Once she quickly learned the rules of any board game, she'd usually beat us, like guessing the identity of a cartoon character in the tile-flipping game "Guess Who?" She also usually became the richest empire-building shark in "Monopoly."

Christmas wasn't Christmas without a few rounds of charades either, and she was always keenly perceptive.

During one of my turns at charades, my task was to act out Noah's Ark.

Oh. My. God …

I showed two fingers. "Two words!"

I nodded. Then I sighed and looked around, completely befuddled. I made smooth waves with my hand.

"Water!" Looking more positive, I nodded slightly but rolled my hands, indicating to keep going. "Ocean!" I shook my head.

No, gotta think of something else … Ahh … yes, maybe …

I held up a finger, reached over and grabbed a decorative basket of artificial fruit on the coffee table. They watched intently, giggling, as I emptied the basket, pointed at it, and signalled word number two.

"Basket?"

I shook my head furiously, extending my hands and stretching them outward, trying to indicate it was something much larger. We were all chortling by now. They had absolutely no idea where I was trying to take them.

Then I noticed Tiger, our fat, old, cowering Tabby, meekly watching our madness from a far corner by the French doors.

Aha!

I hurried over to our submissive beast, secured a stable grip around his belly, lugged him over and plopped him into the basket. The poor kitty immediately bolted, fearing for his life. Hubby and daughter were splitting their guts with hysterical, confused laughter, but I could detect a look in my daughter's eyes that showed something was starting to click.

In desperation, I sat on the floor and started rowing furiously. JP was laughing so hard his eyes were closed.

"NOAH'S ARK!!!" She yelled.

"YES!"

We all laughed until our stomachs hurt and I peed my pants.

✳ ✳ ✳

My daughter grew up to be a force to be reckoned with – fiercely independent, observant and private. She did everything she wanted to do because the rationale she gave was completely incontestable; you just couldn't say no to her.

From age six to ten, her two cousins turned Saturday visits to our house into slumber parties, whenever my brother Fred and his wife Lise came over for supper. After dessert, the girls would scurry down to the "benstant," as my sweetie used to call the basement, and play school. What they were really doing was preparing a manifesto as to why we could not refuse their request to have a sleepover:

1. We have nothing to do the following day.

2. I have extra pyjamas. And there are extra toothbrushes.

3. You won't have to get up early. We will make our own breakfast and clean up after.

4. Dad can drive my cousins back home at 10 a.m. (This relieved Fred and Lise of making the 25-minute road trip on consecutive days.)

With a contract like that, how could we say no?

* * *

I was progressing and becoming more independent, while doing my best to appreciate all the moments of joy with my family.

However, I continued to tell myself that working again just wasn't in my future. But "fate" had a different plan.

17

Resuming My Career?

One day in the spring of 1997, out of the blue, Paul Delparte called me.

His wife Rose, mother of four, had taken excellent care of our little girl when I briefly worked full-time at the Department of the Secretary of State, before my second stroke. Rose also lived right next door to, and was best friends with Debra Laxton, who first made sure our infant daughter was secure with warmth and loving kindness after my first stroke. We were so blessed to have had them in our lives during those times.

"Hey Cathy, a colleague of mine at the Red Cross is looking for a newsletter editor, and I told him about you. He'd really like you to come in for an interview."

"Really?"

I was stupefied, both by Paul's flattery and the presumed

impossibility of taking on this opportunity. I knew I looked and acted normal on the surface to everyone, but I couldn't return to work until I somehow figured out how to better manage the crushing chronic pain, fatigue and invisible sensory disabilities that disturbed every second of my consciousness. Up till then, I figured nobody would ever want to consider hiring a "problem" employee like me.

"Maybe just go to the interview and see how it goes," Paul suggested.

"Sure Paul, that's a good idea," I said, convincing myself aloud. "I really appreciate you thinking of me for this."

A few days later, I stepped over *(careful now, rough terrain)* the breaks in the sidewalk on the giant concourse of the sparkling new Red Cross campus on Alta Vista Drive (now housing Canadian Blood Services) and tried to breathe normally. *Just find the right office, smile, remember the guy's name, shake hands (with your right), and sit down. This is a rehab assignment. You can do this; you just need more practice …*

I don't remember the fellow's name, but he was very kind. The job he described sounded so pleasant, so perfect …

But it was full time. Five days a week.

There was no flexibility in hours of work at the Red Cross, at least for now.

I couldn't even manage full-time hours before the second stroke.

Hanging my head, I murmured apologies to him for his inconvenience, and heard him apologizing for the organization's rigid employment practices. As I started to rise from the chair, half my portfolio dropped all over the floor, but I raised a hand to hold him back from coming to assist me. I would do it my own slow, clumsy way.

"I'll definitely keep you in mind if our hours of work become more flexible," he told me, though we both knew that would never happen. Fighting back tears, I nodded, pulled back the chair, sat and bent over to retrieve the useless samples of my work. I shoved them and the folder into my large shoulder bag and escaped as quickly and painlessly as possible, failing at both.

My heart was in my throat from the defeat, but the experience made me realize that the good thing was that someone had expressed interest in me and my skills. It was up to me to search for the right fit.

I never thanked Paul Delparte enough for nudging me to start thinking that just maybe, there was a way I could return to work again, if someone could reasonably accommodate my differences. So thank you, Paul.

18

Today's Walk

The year was 1996, and our teenage girl was going to French high school next year. After five years of the Botox injections, the markedly decreased foot pain allowed me to figure out the best ways to adapt to the rest of my limitations, and my energy increased significantly.

I made a commitment to go for a walk every day.

I got a pedometer and I kept a log. I continually tried to increase my distance, activity time and number of steps. And I bought the most comfortable, supportive track shoes I could find that would accommodate my brace. Because of the altered proprioception (ability to sense location and movement of parts of one's body) on my right side, buying shoes was always an exhausting nightmare. I needed to walk inside the house with a new pair for at least a week to make sure they weren't pinching my numb foot anywhere, but also flexible enough to securely tighten my larger and stronger left foot, charged with balancing the extra spastic load on my right side. Later, I began to order my shoes online, with free delivery and returns by mail; then I had at least a couple of weeks to test them in the more relaxed reality of my home environment.

Clothing required lots of planning too, and I quickly learned how important it is to have the right equipment or tools to best support my unique needs. I clipped the pedometer onto the waist of my pants and fastened on a waist belt to carry a water bottle to quench my insatiable thirst – a side effect of a medication that calmed the stinging enough to help me fall asleep at night. Since I drank from the bottle so often, I found one I could squeeze and drink from with only my left hand, so that my frequent guzzling would not disturb the improving rhythm I had built up with my right arm and leg. Later, I got myself a water backpack with a convenient nozzle to sip from. The extra weight on my back actually helped balance me better, as well as stand straighter and feel freer, and it also helped me walk more quickly, to "really fly." And now, except on a social occasion requiring smart casual, I wear my water backpack everywhere: to drive, shop, or go out and about.

Today, any form of exertion usually turns me into a sweat-drenched, hot mess; yet, the right side of my neck and arm need to stay covered to soak up the dampness and drafts to help me avoid getting cold and to head off the stinging daggers. Very often, I wear long sleeves with a scarf wrapped around my neck, or else I'm in a lightweight knit cardigan, with my right arm sleeved and the left arm bare, its sleeve slung around my neck and over the right shoulder.

I used to be embarrassed about this, but now, in my mid-sixties, I'm proud to have cornered the market on the hemiparesis look. Also, I always wear a brimmed hat made from material with SPF-50 sunblock, as well as prescription sunglasses to combat photophobia. Sun hurts my eyes, increases dizziness and increases my susceptibility to visual disturbances and migraines.

It hasn't stopped me from being a sun worshipper, though. Whenever the weather permits, I love to "sunbathe" – with only my head kept completely in the shade, and always shielded with a wide-brimmed SPF 50 hat. Fifteen minutes on the right side, another 15 lying on my back and happily, a final roll to the left – just like a rotisserie chicken. Nothing compares to the healing warmth of the sun.

Walking has become my salvation in many ways. There is nothing better than opening the front door first thing in the morning, smelling the cedar hedges and feeling the warmth of the sun on my face, as I mindfully make my way down the steps to the street. Sometimes, I know where I want to go; other times, depending on how I'm feeling, I let the wind carry behind me, or choose to walk into it. On a chilly day, I'll get in the car and turn on the seat heater, and by the time I arrive at my chosen destination, my lower body is all toasty and ready to rock. Either way, it's always an adventure, and every walk is different, even if I go the same way as the day before. On particularly painful days, walks centred around meditation work wonders. I'll count my steps and breathe in (one, two, three, four) and breathe out (one, two, three, four) in sequence. I'll swing my arms back and forth in different positions to work different muscles, in a rhythm to help propel me, or sometimes let them swing limply, with hips turning with each swing – like golfer Dustin Johnson.

I adore walking to the beat of music on Spotify on my trusty iPhone through my hearing aids; with my momentum increasing, I become more spontaneous and joyful. My iPhone doubles as my adventure diary through the (way too many) photos I take, equally due to my lifelong exposure to photography and my obsessive awe when capturing the wonder and beauty of our fragile world.

* * *

For me, every day is an adventure, some kind of a journey, or a "walk," even if I don't literally walk that day.

And that's how my simple "Today's Walk" Facebook posts got started.

I wanted to share my daily journeys with others, because finding joy in the little things in life that are right around us can be so easy to take for granted, yet so surprisingly uplifting when we take a moment to appreciate them.

Perhaps I'll share a photo of something that touched me for its beauty, like a honey bee gathering pollen on a flower. More than anything, "Today's Walk" is my own motivational tool, to remind me that despite my chronic challenges, I am still walking or having some kind of adventure. That in itself brings me joy. And if I give only one other person living with ongoing difficulties some inspiration to help make their day a little easier, I am even happier.

Why do I walk? Because I *can*.

Fortunately, I have not spent much time in a wheelchair, but long enough to understand how irrevocably it can affect one's mobility. Every day, my own mobility issues cloud my mind, threaten my independence, remind me of its fragility, and impel me to work as hard as I can so that I can continue to enjoy my life as freely as possible.

So I walk. For me, walking is a blessing. When I walk, I enjoy every bit of life I can see, hear, taste and smell.

Because I *can*. And I love nature.

I take photos of huge yellow sunflowers. A Cooper's hawk preying on a rodent in a neighbouring tree. Gleeful children sliding down a steep front-yard toboggan hill with their Daddy guarding them from careening into the street, while holding a Foster's beer in one mittened hand. A white sandy beach kissed by turquoise waters on a dead coral reef. Evergreens dripping with melting snow …

I can trace my love of nature back to my early years. My happiest childhood memories come from one of our summer family-camping trips to the formerly orchard-rich (and now tragically fire-ravaged) Okanagan Valley in British Columbia, when I was seven years old. This was also when I discovered the joy of eating peaches.

We visited a peach orchard in the warm sunshine, the air ripe with spicy sweet scents of the fruit. I remember climbing up a ladder placed against one of the loaded trees, reaching out and snapping off a huge, orangey-red ball the size of a small grapefruit and chomping through the fuzz into its sweet, juicy succulence, its thick warm liquid running down my chin. That is partly how I acquired my reverence for the infinitesimal powers of the sun as the fire that sparks life on this spinning ball of earth and water, orbiting around it in the universe. This led me to a fascination with origins: astrology, Tarot cards and a keen interest in archaeology, anthropology and other mysteries of past societies. Now I am both enthralled and horrified by climate change and the devastation of the increasingly violent and unpredictable winds, torrential rains, floods, fires, and unbearable heat and cold vortexes that are threatening our survival. I am not a religious person, but I do feel a spiritual responsibility to try to do whatever I can to help our environment – like an armchair Earth Mother.

As a young girl, I had fleeting thoughts that someday I'd like to be a naturalist or park ranger, like Ranger Smith on *Yogi Bear*. Or maybe I would dig up key artefacts leading to a fuller understanding of the origins and evolution of humanity, like paleoanthropologist and archaeologist, Dr. Louis Leakey, with his groundbreaking discoveries at Olduvai Gorge in Tanzania. But these were merely fanciful ideas.

My darling daughter awarded me the nickname "Goulet," after Will Ferrell's hilarious "Nature, Goulet" skits on Saturday Night Live. In them, Ferrell is doing a playful impersonation of Canadian/American entertainer Robert Goulet, well-known as a debonair and often overly flamboyant character. (Check it out on YouTube.) That's me alright. I'm definitely a Goulet.

People I pass by usually return my smile, nod or greeting, even when I'm struggling. Always dressed to enjoy a fun adventure, I try not to watch my feet and keep my pace determined, and during pandemic times, smiling eyes peeking over facemasks would often meet mine first. Smiles are so healing.

I try to walk every day, and go farther and longer. A walk will often include taking short breaks at one or two bus stops or on park benches. I'll locate my sitz bones: the sweet spot that helps lengthen my spine and centre my pelvis, breathe deeply, assess what's bothering me most and then get on with the best way to keep moving. Sometimes I'll use my own little yogic walking mantras like "Do Dirty DJ" (lope like golfer Dustin Johnson), "Just Do It" (former Nike slogan) or "Keep Diggin" (a Mr. Sub commercial where a Mafia Don is forcing a skinny thief of microwave ovens to dig his own grave). Humour is so healing. When I laugh, nothing hurts.

19

A Token Appointment:
Justice from Justice

It took about a year from the time I made the conscious decision to try to restart my career for me to land the most ideal dream job I could imagine.

By 1996, I had regained so much resilience since the Botox injections had reduced my pain enough to lessen my brain's never-ending preoccupation with fight or flight and to expand past short-term, basic thinking. We had a family meeting and agreed that it would be good for me to get out there to attempt another reboot, albeit with conditions.

I could not work full time. I needed to be up-front about my disabilities, since they were mostly invisible. This could be a huge turn-off for any prospective employer, since the last thing any manager wants to do is take on a problem employee with a potential "liability" or invest in someone who might produce less because of their "condition." People with disabilities or chronic issues have to work harder at everything.

I was fortunate to live in Canada's capital because of its rich, federal public service communications environment. I loved my short stint as a freelance writer with several fascinating departments; however, self-employment required more "cold-calls" and paper-work stress, and the biggest drawback of all: no pension. Now, I needed stability and security, not just financially, but also in my regular day-to-day routine. I needed an environment where I would be able to factor in all the extra energy requirements just to make it into the office, work all day (with perhaps a 20-minute meditative lie-down somewhere quiet, like in a nurse's office, maybe?), then make it back home in one piece. And that's a hard sell for a com-munications gig, which often involves last-minute publication deadlines, media, political and public relations crises.

With my previous experience, the federal public service was the only environment I targeted because it was officially committed to respecting differences and increasing diversity.

Regardless, I figured three days a week would be my maximum threshold, at least to start. So I sent an application letter and resume, along with a few samples of my work, to more than a dozen big bosses of communications in departments I thought might be a good fit.

But after a month, no response.

I had to rethink my strategy.

"You may remember my recent letter, where I expressed interest in working three days per week," my follow-up letter began. "After careful consideration, I would be interested in a four-day work week at the office, with the fifth day at home."

I got only one call back, from Karen Laughlin, Director General of Communications at the Department of Justice.

And it changed my life.

I became the editor of the department's employee newsletter, entitled *inter pares* (Latin for "among equals"). I would be replacing local author Clive Doucet, who had just won a seat in the City of Ottawa election as a counsellor for the Capital Ward. And the position was mid-level! Ha! Back in 1976, when I was slogging it out at Health Canada as a secretary in media relations, I remember gazing mournfully at the press officers and thinking that without a degree, I could never do what they did. Now, after everything I had gone through, I was getting this opportunity!

For the interview, I wore moss-green, cotton pants with a smart-looking, matching angular woven top. My outfit concealed my brace because I didn't want anyone to see it right away. Since wearing the brace, I had noticed that some people release expressions of surprise, discomfort or even a hint of aversion upon first seeing it. And for a prospective employer, I feared it could potentially generate false perceptions, or distract them with sympathy and therefore, concerns about my capabilities.

"I'll be honest with you, it wasn't your writing that impressed me," Karen told me. "It's that you have disabilities, and we need to help you get back into the workforce. I've worked with Terry Fox, so I have some understanding about the difficulties you face."

Essentially, she was telling me that I would be a "token" hire, but even though that term can sound a bit negative, I didn't see it that way. Karen was telling me that she wanted to give me rights and opportunities that I could have been denied.

"Here's what I can offer you," she continued. "We'll hire you as a full-time, term employee for the first three months, so you can get established, and then you can go down to a four-day work week."

I was smiling and nodding before she finished talking. "Yes!" I chirped. "That would be perfect!"

Karen smiled, then looked down, squirmed in her chair ever so slightly and directed a somewhat uneasy expression my way.

"I know I'm not supposed to ask you this, and you don't have to answer, vis-a-vis your right to privacy," she began, knowing from my letter that I'd had two strokes, "But what are your disabilities?

Yay! She realizes that appearing "normal" doesn't mean you're like everybody else …

"I used to be right-handed, but now I'm left-handed, and I wear a brace on my right leg."

She smiled, got up and shook my right hand.

"Welcome aboard, Cathy."

* * *

My first day was November 10, 1997. Perfect. November 11 was Remembrance Day, and a statutory holiday. This would allow me to attack full force on "Day One" at Justice, fully suited up, firing with all my guns, and the next day I would lie back, lick my wounds, and contemplate all the ways I would learn how to adapt to my new environment in order to get the job done.

That was the scariest part. Could I pull it off?

Jean-Pierre and I drove downtown together. I also got a bus pass that said, "I Cannot Stand on a Moving Bus." We arrived at the office and returned home as early as we could, to ease traffic strains. His office, at Place de Ville, was just across the Sparks Street Mall from mine. Sweet. The worries of commuting were reduced to weathering my chauffeur's heavy foot and sporadic rants whenever he encountered automotive idiots. Understood and expected. I would try hard to refrain from being a backseat driver.

At first, JP dropped me off in front of the original Justice Building at the western frontier of Parliament Hill, next to the Supreme Court of Canada. A month later, the Department moved across Wellington Street to the newly renovated East Memorial Building. But what a privilege it had been for me to work in the original building – this spectacular, gothic-inspired, historic base of Canada's first lawmakers at the time of Confederation, if even for such a short time.

On my first day, I arrived at Clive Doucet's former office at 8:00 a.m. and was greeted by Line Routhier, the communications department's electronic word-processing wizard. Always working on several projects at one time, Line flawlessly inputted texts, charts, photos, illustrations and codings that would become bilingual Justice publications, as well as internal directives and communication to roughly 5,000 staff across Canada. She was the only one around when I arrived, as her station was just outside my office. Over the years, we worked as a tag team on a wide array of products and became very close colleagues.

Fortunately, my return to the workforce came at a time when Justice had just started to use email – less than a year before my arrival. Email was completely foreign to me, but I was not too far behind everyone else. Line expertly tutored me and showed me tricks to fix my temperamental office printer. She was always cheerful, took quiet satisfaction in her efficiency, and thrived on solving every technological issue and meeting every deadline thrown her way when she was producing the Department's messaging products. The more pressure in production, the more focussed she became.

* * *

At first, it felt as if I was slowly being sucked down into a thick, swirling miasma. *How long will it take for everyone to realize that I don't have a clue what I'm doing? I've had to bail from jobs so early, so many times before … how long will it take this time around?*

On the Sunday after my first two-day week, I brought JP into the office with me for support. I wanted to settle in, read, and try to ground myself and my thoughts, and at the very least, figure out what I needed to focus on to survive the next five-day week. Not just mentally, but physically. *Five days, for three whole months … WTF were you thinking?*

I wandered around the office with a grey, insidious feeling of panic, pawing through the hanging files in the bottom drawer of my desk, reading completely nonsensical emails, and thinking, *What have you gotten yourself into? Marie-Claire is hoping that the first issue of inter pares comes out BEFORE Christmas … how am I going to make that happen?*

I hung in for more than a decade, though, and thrived. I even got promoted to my level of incompetence, ha ha. More on that later.

My first manager, the impeccably polite and refined Marie-Claire Wallace, had been a senior journalist at *Le Droit,* Ottawa's French-language newspaper. As Justice's director of publications, she aspired to perfection in the craft of all things written in both official languages.

"Tomorrow, I'll take you around the fourth floor and introduce you to everyone," she told me on my first Monday.

I was happy to get the advance notice. The next day, I walked into the office wearing my denim shirtdress, exposing the flat desert boots that fit over my braced leg. This was not to signal that I was disabled, but rather, *differently* abled. (For example, whenever I use a cane equipped with a retractable ice pick to navigate frozen or rough terrain in winter, it instantly signals that I have a mobility issue, and that a bit more space to navigate might be a good idea. The accommodative response from the visual cue to others then becomes instinctive, and as the waters gently part for me with no questions asked, I slog forward with a quick nod and a thankful smile.)

My new office mates all seemed delighted to meet me, and I caught a few eye flickers downwards. One person asked if I had an injury. I replied that I'd had a stroke. As her eyes widened, I smiled and said "but I'm still walking and talking," and that was good enough for me and the communications gang.

When I was in social situations, particularly when meeting someone for the first time, or, as another example, introducing myself when I was bringing my daughter to a playgroup when she was younger, I had this terribly anxious habit of blurting out, "I'm Cathy Allard, and I've had two strokes." I was terrified that the odd hitch in my gait or periodic jerking to keep my balance might lead a stranger to perceive me to be a drunkard or a druggie. I also worried about being asked or expected to participate in some process or activity that would not be safe for me to attempt, especially if I'd never tried to do it before.

* * *

When Pierre Trudeau died on September 28, 2000, the Communications branch went into a frenzy to prepare a tribute to the former Minister of Justice who had gone on to become Prime Minister.

Marie-Claire was a member of the National Press Club, a couple of blocks up the hill from us. That day, she bustled back to our office after lunch at the Press Club, carrying a large brown envelope and appearing unusually excited. Someone had given her something special.

She carefully extracted two very rare, 11 x 14-inch glossy photos of Monsieur Trudeau in his famous "gunslinger" pose, taken by renowned American portrait photographer David Montgomery. This particular photo was used in the 1979 election campaign, but very few prints were ever produced. It shows Trudeau leaning against the carved wood wall in his House of Commons office, posing with his fingers tucked in the belt of his brown corduroy pants, his face quietly determined, as if to say "bring it on." It was an amazingly intimate capture.

"The photographer is a friend of mine," she gushed.

"Oh wow!" I blurted, "I would just love to have one of those!"

Marie-Claire hesitated, wondering a moment. Then she nodded happily, realizing how big a fan I was. After all, as an Anglophone from British Columbia who, after moving to Ottawa, learned to speak French remarkably well … I was living proof of how the *Official Languages Act* was meant to work.

So, Marie-Claire gave me one of those portraits and today, "Pierre" holds a place of honour mounted on the wall in our basement, next to the late painter Ben Babelowsky's rendition of the original Justice Building, where I enjoyed working for all of one month. Sweet memories!

* * *

I made quite a few silly mistakes early on. I received a kind phone call of rebuke from our Northwest Territories regional office for spelling Iqaluit "Iqualuit" in the first issue of *inter pares*.

My most shameful boo-boo as the editor of *inter pares* occurred when I had tightened up a voluminous article written by Daniel Bellemare, our powerful Deputy Attorney General of Canada, chronicling his personal audience with the late great Nelson Mandela. Editing his tome was fine in itself, but I worried about how the article and photos would fit the allotted space in print, so I sent my unapproved shortened text and photos off for a quick mock-up before forwarding the condensed text to Monsieur Bellemare for his final approval.

Coincidentally, when he was in Marie-Claire's office to discuss an unrelated matter, the deputy AG's sharp eyes picked out the mock-up on Marie-Claire's desk, already laid out before he had approved the shortened copy. And as you might guess, not knowing it was merely a mock-up, he exploded.

Most of us were terrified by the power and the authority he wielded. Lucky for me though, I got off easy, receiving only the wrath of my immediate boss.

Time heals nearly all wounds, though. Monsieur Bellemare and I bumped into each other many years later, at Bruyère Foot Specialists (as many of us seniors now need professionals to buzz-saw our hardened calluses and chunky toenails off our feet), and we enjoyed a friendly chat. He told me he had retired, and his love of all things legal had been replaced by a passion for antiques.

Later in my job at the Justice Department, I found myself producing the print version of *inter pares* while helping develop content, writing and editing for our brand-new weekly electronic employee news bulletin called *JustInfo,* which the fabulous Line Routhier coded, entered and published without fail, every Friday morning. It was short, concise (unlike my own writing) and complete with hyperlinks for further details.

When it became clear that the articles of *inter pares* could be easily incorporated into *JustInfo,* the print edition was put to rest, thus saving a few more trees.

I retired in 2009, just before the onslaught of social media. Lucky me.

* * *

It was an honour for me to work with and cover the amazing achievements of Justice's tireless staff. Its lawyers certainly aren't in the federal public service for the money; in private industry, they could rake in probably three times as much dough. Justice attorneys are idealistic, socially conscious and dedicated to improving our rights and freedoms within the confines of our laws.

* * *

One of my biggest thrills was interviewing then-Minister of Justice Irwin Cotler in his House of Commons office in 2004. An international human rights lawyer and icon for peace and justice, Mr. Cotler has been cited as "a scholar and advocate of international stature." His achievements while Minister of Justice included crafting the *Civil Marriage Act,* the first-ever legislation to grant marriage equality to gays and lesbians. He also initiated the first-ever law in Canada on human trafficking and introduced our first national initiative against racism and hate. He also overturned more wrongful convictions in one year than any previous Minister of Justice.

Another contribution that brings me pride was my work to organize a tribute commemorating the unveiling of a monument to Henriette Bourque, the first female lawyer to work at the Justice Department, from 1939 to 1949. Her son, Dr. Pierre Bourque, a neurologist at the Ottawa Hospital, was delighted to attend the ceremony, and I was both surprised and delighted to receive a letter of appreciation from then-Deputy Minister Morris Rosenberg for my efforts.

Perhaps the most gratifying experience during my decade at Justice was my time as a volunteer with the Deputy Minister's Advisory Committee on Persons with Disabilities (ACPD). Its members, many of whom were senior Justice executives, were delighted to have a representative from internal communications to help spread the word about their work and give them guidance from a communications perspective.

Justice lawyer Carole Théberge, Chair of the ACPD, also had a personal stake in the Committee. This cheerful woman who was profoundly hard of hearing quietly understood and accepted the extra difficulties that people with disabilities have in representing themselves on an even keel with "The Others" (my affectionate phraseology – not Carole's), not to mention integrating themselves. She regularly organized ad hoc presentations from differently abled colleagues employed in other government departments to talk about issues they were working on. I will never forget the tiny, bespectacled attorney who floated into the conference room one day and quickly seated herself, with an almost invisible assistant right behind her.

She had no arms.

Her assistant placed a report in front of her. Carole quickly introduced her, and she greeted everyone with a pleasant smile, efficient and all business.

She outlined the changes she was helping her department make to better accommodate different people like us, so that we could fit in as seamlessly as possible and maximize our performance …

She had no arms. She was turning the pages with her teeth.

Between breaths. Continuing her discourse.

Hardly a pause.

How could she do that? How did she ever become a lawyer?

Now there was a woman with determination.

20

Foot Reconstruction

My right foot continued to deteriorate. When muscles stop functioning and cease to move, they tighten up and begin to atrophy. My toes were curling up. And the Botox injections had started to lose their effectiveness, as I had been warned.

In 2000, I had even started to wear a customized night brace to try to keep my right foot straight while I slept. Or tried to sleep.

Dr. Anna McCormick, the tiny and cheerful pediatric muscular-dystrophy specialist who had been keeping my foot looser and more comfortable in the daytime brace with the Botox injections, took off her gloves one day after finishing the routine two or three excruciating stabs, and looking contemplative, asked me a surprising question.

"How would you feel about having surgery to straighten out your foot?" My eyes widened and she nodded. "Maybe it's time we start thinking about it."

"Oh yes, that would be wonderful! Sign me up!"

She smiled at my enthusiasm. "This would be major surgery though," she cautioned. "It would involve a lengthy recovery period. But you're young and otherwise in good health, and I think you'd do very well. You might not even need to wear the brace anymore."

My eyes widened. "REALLY?"

She nodded. "I think there's a very good possibility. So, if you agree, I'd like to refer you to Jacques Brunet; he's an amazing orthopedic surgeon, and I really think he could help you. It'll take a year just to get in to see him for a consult, though."

"I don't care how long it takes." I would do anything for the chance to rid myself of dragging what felt like an iron ball on a chain – an impediment that bit into me with every step, and now, with every turn in bed. "Please make the referral."

⋆ ⋆ ⋆

Dr. Brunet was a pleasant man of few words. After a short examination and a request to see me walk back and forth, he smiled and sat down in front of me.

"Okay, we're going to reconstruct your foot using tendon transfers and extensions," he told me. "When we do a transfer, we move the attached tendon over to another part of the foot to help it function better." Then he smiled. "To do tendon extensions, we make long, zed-shaped 'Zorro' cuts," he added, making a playful motion of the letter Z with his index finger, as if he was going to relish creating them.

"After the surgery, your leg will be casted up to your knee. The leg should be kept raised as much as possible, and you cannot put any weight on it for six weeks."

"Six weeks in bed?"

"Pretty much, yes. To get out of bed and use the bathroom, you will need to use crutches." He consulted my file. "You live in a two-storey house, right?" I nodded, and he continued. "You'll have to go up and down the stairs on your butt, and use a wheelchair to get around downstairs. I understand your daughter is self-sufficient, and your husband is very supportive?"

"Oh yes. She's studying in Toronto, and Jean-Pierre is amazing."

"That's great," he said. "I should also mention that because your leg will be immobilized for such a long time, you will have to inject yourself with blood thinners every day, but it's quite easy; you don't need to find a vein. You don't have an aversion to needles, do you?"

"After Botox? Naaahhh … " That brought a little chuckle.

"All right, we'll get you scheduled then. It'll probably be in February."

"Could you please write the name of the procedures down for me?"

He nodded and cheerfully wrote them down. "You won't find this on the internet though," he told me.

We shook hands, I thanked him, and the deed was done on Valentine's Day, 2002.

* * *

After waking up in the recovery room and being greeted by a nurse, I carefully peeled the sheet away to get a look at the cast. A small gasp escaped from my lips.

"Yikes!"

The fat, heavy white cast enveloped the entire lower leg and opened up at the toes, revealing the top of a huge, black spike defiantly protruding nearly an inch out of the top of my big toe.

It looked like something out of *Frankenstein!*

I was told everything went well though, and I was sent home after two nights.

Six weeks was indeed a very long time to be confined at home in bed, but it went surprisingly quickly. Every morning I would haul myself to the ensuite on the crutches, do my business and shoot myself up with the blood thinner. Before JP left for the office, he brought me a tray with yogurt, fruit, coffee and the newspaper, along with a paper bag full of surprises for lunch. I usually read all the news, did all the puzzles on the crossword page, then read a book and watched *The Price is Right* with good ol' Bob Barker. My neighbours were wonderful too; they dropped in for the odd visit or gave JP a break and brought lunch. I actually lost 20 pounds and got pretty fit too, hoisting myself ass-backwards up and down the stairs and into the wheelchair at least once a day.

After the initial six weeks, it was back to the hospital to have the cast cut open with a power saw, removed and examined by "Foot Magician" Jacques Brunet.

A thick black line of huge, criss-crossing stitches ran halfway down inside my lower leg and curled halfway past the inside of the foot. The tortured big toe was slashed with the same black sutures right down the middle to the base of the toenail, buttressed by the brutal black spike spearing out through the top.

"Looks really good," Dr. Brunet assured me.

"Well I'm glad you think so – it looks like I'm in a *Frankenstein* movie!"

"The marks from your stitches should actually fade pretty quickly," he told me with a hint of a smile. "Now, I see you brought the crutches; that's good. You can start using them now. The new cast we're putting on today will be lighter and have a solid piece added to the heel for more protection and stability, but still, it's very important not to put any weight on that foot. Take another two weeks to get used to using your crutches at home with your right knee bent, and foot raised behind you, off the floor. After that, you can go back to work, using the crutches for another week. We'll see you again in three weeks, remove the cast and see where you're at. You should be ready to start physiotherapy by then. Any questions?"

"Nope. Sounds great!" It was all I could do not to ask him if he thought I would be able to walk again without the cursed brace, but I knew it was too soon. In the meantime, I would do everything he asked, short of biting off my silly big toe.

* * *

The Department of Justice was incredibly supportive throughout my absence, assigning others to pick up the slack, as I had often done for them. When I returned to work all casted and crutched, most of my colleagues could not help gasping the first time they saw me, rattled by what they perceived to be my grave misfortune.

Including Deputy Minister Morris Rosenberg.

He happened to be in his reception lobby, paper in hand, deep in discussion with his executive assistant, when I clomped through the glass entryway in front of them, clinging to an urgent document they were expecting.

His gaze froze on me.

"What happened to you?"

"Oh, no worries," I said, grinning sheepishly while his assistant Philomena Arruda took the paper from me. "It's all good – it was a planned intervention."

With a nod and a "see you later," signifying that it was not my intention to interrupt them, I turned myself around with the crutches and clippety-clopped back to my office.

* * *

A week later, back at the Ottawa hospital, Dr. Brunet removed the cast and examined his work.

"Okay, looks good. We can remove the pin now," he said to his attending technician, referring to the giant spike protruding from my big toe. Surprisingly, despite my stomach curdling, it didn't hurt at all, and there was hardly any bleeding. A simple band-aid was applied, and I was told to keep one on for a few days.

"Everything looks perfect," he said, looking pleased. "Are you ready to start physio now?"

"Oh yes."

"Good." He scratched his head, gathering his thoughts. "Now, you should continue to use the crutches, but you can start putting light weight on your foot, at least until your first physiotherapy appointment. I'll want you to go to the Cleave Clinic, twice a week. They're on Metcalfe Street."

"C-L-E-A-V-E?" I repeated.

"Yes, the Cleave Physiotherapy and Sports Injury Clinic. I really like them; they're very good at this sort of thing." He scribbled out a prescription and gave it to Jean-Pierre. "Bring this along with you on your first visit, and they'll take good care of you." He stood back, smiling slightly. "Any questions?"

I couldn't wait any longer. "So, do you think I can go South this winter and throw my brace into the ocean?"

"Oh yes," he said, smiling. "It looks very good. And call my office to set up a follow-up appointment for about a month from now."

Jean-Pierre and I floated all the way home.

* * *

A few days later, JP spotted me as I crutched up the five steep, concrete stairs of the run-down, crumbling six-story office building on Metcalfe Street that housed Cleave Physiotherapy.

And who was the first person who crossed my path as I bumbled through the front door?

The Great Graham Curryer … Past Bringer of Botox.

"Hey – I heard you were coming in this morning!" He gestured toward my foot, looking so delighted he was almost bouncing. "This is fantastic!"

"Yeah, I know, Graham! So good to see you again! You work here now?"

"Yeah, and I've also started my own business. Come drop by my cubicle after your physio, and we can chat for a minute if there's time."

That day was the last time I saw him.

My gratitude toward this kind, innovative healthcare professional was overshadowed by horror and dismay, upon learning that he took his own life on December 29, 2011. He was only 44 years old.

21

Promotions, More Surgeries & Other Ills

You may recall my stint as a junior writer/editor at Secretary of State, where I came up with the phrase "Independence – That's Living" for a poster promoting what became International Day for Persons with Disabilities, proclaimed by the United Nations on December 3, 1992. All federal public service departments now funnelled their disability-awareness activities to coincide with and celebrate the "Big Day."

Now working for the Justice Department, I took it upon myself to organize an exhibition in the foyer of the East Memorial Building, which backed onto the Sparks Street pedestrian mall. The exhibition consisted of several tables and stations staffed by knowledgeable people, whose mission was to highlight the variety of ways that people with disabilities can increase their independence.

Think of the late theoretical physicist, cosmologist and author

Stephen Hawking, who used a keyboard in his wheelchair equipped with a tiny gear he could control with one gnarled finger, both to speak and write out volumes of his brain's genius. Also consider braille, sign language, hearing aids and closed-captioning for TV shows or public presentations, as well as braces, canes, motorized wheelchairs, and artificial limbs – even some with moveable hands and fingers. These are only a few examples that just scratch the surface of what's available – but it can take supreme efforts from those who need supports just to figure out what's available and then find a "wizard" to adapt it to their specific requirements. The increased expense and complexity required to craft the appropriate devices can be mind-boggling and simply out of reach for many people with disabilities.

As a simple example, let's say you've found the perfect wheelchair, and you want to go back to work. However, you can't make it to the interview for that perfect job because the building has no lowered curbs to allow your wheelchair to get into the building. That's a readily visible example of a workplace accessibility issue.

Justice's Occupational Health and Safety (OH&S) Division, led by the marvellous Bea Hertz, was ahead of its time in promoting awareness and compliance with many complex accommodations issues that have since become almost standard practice in schools, workplaces and other institutions nowadays.

For example, take the growing requirement that public places be scent-free. The perfume you adore can cause migraines, nausea, breathing problems and even anaphylactic reactions in others. My brother, Fred Roberts, once on a flight from Ottawa to Vancouver via Calgary, became so violently ill from inhaling a passenger's perfume from the seat behind him that he was escorted off the plane in Calgary and sent to a hotel to recover. For me, lavender, an herb heavily used in spa and relaxation products, causes migraine vomit-fests that shutter me in a dark room for a couple of days before I can keep anything down. Just the smell of peanut butter or seafood can send others into anaphylaxis.

Fires and fire drills in office towers pose what may seem like insurmountable safety concerns for people with disabilities. If the elevators are disabled, how does someone with mobility issues make it down the stairwell? At Justice, OH&S secured me a mechanical "caterpillar" that could crawl down stairs with me belted into it, controlled by one person down below and another up behind me.

The International Day of Persons With Disabilities exhibit on December 3, 2005, included the participation of a couple of Assistant Deputy Ministers and was well received by staff. Monique Collette, a senior executive who often collaborated with the ACPD, approached me soon after.

"I think you have qualities that would make you a terrific executive," she gushed. "If you agree, I'd be delighted to sponsor you for the EX training program."

For once, I was so taken by surprise that I was speechless.

"Wow, thank you Monique," I finally breathed, "I feel so honoured … but I don't know if I could handle it … how demanding is it?"

As Monique told me a little bit about the training program, all

I could think was *Ohhh, damn … this is SO tempting … could be so wonderful … but I know I can't even think about it … it's all I can do to fit in, as it is … my family already supports me so much … and I have to be able to give back …*

"Think about it for a while, and let me know," Monique suggested. "I think you'd be amazing."

I soon declined, though. Deep down, I knew I wouldn't be able to handle it physically. My family was too important to me to rock the boat any further. Life was already better than I ever imagined it could be because of the sacrifices they made every day to allow me to enjoy working again. I didn't do heavy housework or make meals anymore, except on weekends; my biggest priorities were to get myself dressed, make it to the office, and put in a full day's work without doing anything too stupid.

* * *

The Communications Branch inevitably went through a reorganization and created an Internal Communications Team. Susan Gardner-Barclay became my new director. She was intelligent and supportive, with high expectations. We underwent a physical office move, and I ended up kitty-corner to Suesan Saville, another communications director at that time. The two Su(e)sans inspired me and gave me plenty of creative management opportunities. When our team leader, Karen Allen, went on maternity leave, I enjoyed a short acting assignment in her role. I even hired a few short-term employees, including a terrific writer, Season Osborne, who later published a Canadian Arctic history book entitled *In the Shadow of the Pole: An Early History of Arctic Expeditions, 1871 –1912,*

Dundurn Press, 2013.

Not long after, Virginia McRae, an attorney heading up the Family Law Division who was recently involved with the Disabilities Committee, let me know that John Sims, our Deputy Minister of Justice, had asked her to become Director General of a new unit that would report directly to him, and they would need a senior communications officer. Would I be interested in this new position?

I didn't hesitate for a second. I loved Virginia. She was the most supportive, appreciative and hands-off boss who knew how to empower her employees. Her Executive Assistant, Dianne Charlebois, was also amazing. Virginia left hand-written thank-you notes. And DM John Sims was known for randomly popping into anyone's office on the way into his own, first thing in the morning, just to say hi and ask how you were doing.

I couldn't believe that in 2005, I had exceeded my wildest dreams.

After I first became ill, I managed to eke out some publishing experience on my own, in lieu of a degree in journalism. I also benefitted from networking with friends. And then, after sorting out my biggest obstacles as a result of the second stroke, I believe I reached out far enough to be considered for a token appointment.

I welcomed Karen Laughlin giving me any opportunity of a tryout, since I wasn't even sure if I could do it myself.

She understood the need for me to figure out my own personal logistics and prove myself in a full-time, three-month trial before Justice took me on with the four-day week. That was a fair deal, and it's one way responsible employers can try to integrate staffing quotas for "under-represented" individuals, because they can need more time and effort to settle in and do things differently. I feel extremely blessed to have had such cutting-edge rehabilitation, not just once, but twice, and I also appreciate that many other people in my situation do not get such timely care or appropriate support from family, friends and the healthcare sector. I was also probably fast-tracked into rehabilitation because I was a young mother.

Another mom who took my rehab bed at Saint-Vincent Hospital was not as fortunate as I had been. She had a brain bleed that left her with a totally useless arm. She also had two little boys, and her marriage broke up. Research has indicated that the risk of divorce is much higher when the wife gets sick. For example, when a woman has surgery for a brain tumour, almost 80 per cent of their partners leave them within the first year.[1]

People with disabilities often don't have access to the support or the tools they need to advocate for themselves, even for the most basic health care.

And yes, my education and professional skills may have been under par, but again, because I still had some writing skills with a bit of marketing experience, I figured out how to become my own advocate. It can be extremely difficult for a person with disabilities to apply for a job because their confidence already sucks, and they have such limited extra bandwidth to display themselves in a way in which the employer will not feel overly uncomfortable. Managers themselves are terrified to ask too many questions, for fear of being

---

[1] *Invisible: How Young Women With Serious Health Issues Navigate Work, Relationships, and the Pressure to Seem Just Fine*, Michele Lent Hirsch, 2018. Beacon Press.

accused of discrimination. But employers are not mind readers, either. I was forced to talk about my own issues because they were, for the most part, invisible.

I knew I would be ending my career in a wonderful spot, even though it took me a couple of weeks to be able to pronounce where I had been promoted to. It was a mouthful: Strategic Planning and Performance Management (SPPM).

* * *

At age 50, I began to recognize that my working days would soon be coming to an end.

One morning, I happened to meet up with my big boss Virginia McRae, now ADM of Corporate Affairs, at the elevator on our way to a meeting, holding my familiar-to-everyone red metal coffee cup from Prague, adorned with cartoon cats, forever filled with water to manage my dry mouth issues.

I thought the light smile on Virginia's face was for the crazy cartoon cats on my bright red mug, but she leaned closer and murmured, "Cathy, you have a toilet paper tail."

I was SO embarrassed!

"Here, give me your cup," she said softly, taking it from me. "I'll bring it to the meeting while you go get yourself sorted out."

Managing my own shit below the waist was literally becoming harder and harder. In addition to the two foot surgeries, I needed more time off work for a hysterectomy and then an internal hemorrhoidectomy to arrest heavy bleeding from both ends. Constipation had been a problem for me since my late teens, and after the strokes, it became exhausting and horrific.

Dr. Luc Rochon, the gastrointestinal specialist who referred me for the surgery after a colonoscopy, gave me some good advice.

"You should always use moist baby wipes down there."

Dr. Benoit St-Jean, the gifted surgeon at Montfort Hospital who repaired my internal tear, told me I was the fourth-worst case he'd ever seen. I shocked myself just as much as him when I grasped his hand and just said, "thank you."

Dr. David McCoubrey of Montfort Hospital also came through with a brilliant partial hysterectomy. A large orange-sized fibroid was growing inside my uterus, turning my monthly periods into eight-day bloody deluges. He told me the surgery had been a bit difficult, but he was able to successfully remove everything through the vagina, leaving the ovaries intact. I was on cloud nine – no incision, no periods and no instant menopause! One fantastic deal!!

However, unbeknownst to me at the time, these two surgeries, combined with chronic constipation and the scars from the difficult birth all contributed to a condition now more commonly known as pelvic prolapse. More common with women than men, pelvic prolapse is essentially a weakened core; it can affect your ability to hold your body upright, go to the bathroom properly or have sex without pain. It can also cause incontinence and recurrent urinary tract infections or UTIs, which hurt like the bejeezus and ultimately cause kidney damage, unless treated with antibiotics. My evil husband often jokes, "Oh no, not another DUI, or is it an IUD, gee – what the heck you got down there?" I try hard not to laugh, because laughing can make me pee, which with a UTI, stings like crazy.

In the meantime, horrific migraines, tied to my hormonal cycles, continued to plague me. Often I'd wake up with a hideous headache and pop an Imitrex before leaving for work.

For a long time, Imitrex was my miracle drug; it quickly quelled the nausea and unbearable lights and sounds. But sometimes, I'd end up tossing my cookies in the ladies room about an hour after arriving at the office anyway, and JP would have to pick me up and ferry me back to a dark room back home.

By 2006, chronic pain now crawled all over me all the time, like mad leeches. Even after a good day at the office, my stronger left side often raged at me for instinctively bearing the brunt of its efforts to support the weaker right side. This led to extra fatigue, which always led to more stinging and burning. By the time we were exiting the Queensway at Montreal Road and almost back home, my mouth was already watering for that blissful triple shot of Johnnie Walker on the rocks, along with a tasty puff of weed to relax everything … just numb everything …

I feared that chronic pain risked turning me into a raging alcoholic and drug addict.

One Friday, near the end of a heavy period (before the hysterectomy), and after another gruelling day, my thirst for scotch was insatiable. I also enjoyed a toke while setting up the Scrabble board for a round while Jean-Pierre put dinner together. I hurt all over, felt so spent, so needy for nothing but numbness. Jean-Pierre brought me the beloved glass, ahhh, Johnnie … and another icy gulp of liquid gold caressed my tongue and throat. Ahhhh …

After a while, I felt less pain, but woosh, I was so whacked out.

I looked at my wooden letter tiles. The letters were a jumble. They made no words, no sense at all …

Ahhh … you're just … so, so tired … just find a three-letter word, then. OK. P-A-N …

What word was it again? … oh yeah … starts with P …

So … pick up the P …

But my hands stayed in my lap. Then my heart leapt into my throat.

Am I having another stroke?

Nah … don't really think so … just wanna go to sleep …

"I don't feel like playing anymore," I mumbled. I just wanted to go to bed. He stared at me, flabbergasted as I started to rise and then just crumpled gently to the floor, like a ragdoll.

"Ohmygod, Cathy!" JP was on the floor in a flash, holding me. "What – are you having another stroke?"

"No, no … I don't think so … I just feel so weak … it's probably just that my period's so heavy …"

"Hmmm. You do look really pale," he said, assessing me. But I could tell he wasn't satisfied.

"It's just that – if it's a stroke, the sooner you get to the hospital, the better … "

I let go of a big sigh. The very last thing I wanted to do was go to the hospital. But he was right. I wasn't sure.

"Okay, call Telehealth and talk to a nurse."

The nurse agreed that we should call an ambulance so that a proper assessment could be made. I begrudgingly went along with it, if only for our peace of mind, since I appreciated the life-and-death importance of seeking immediate attention after a stroke, but I insisted on walking to the ambulance and being strapped onto the gurney only once inside. I wanted to minimize hysterical neighbourhood scrutiny.

Given that I lay on the gurney in the hospital's ambulance dumping ground for two hours, I became 100 per cent certain that they'd agree that it was not a stroke, but rather 100 per cent substance abuse.

I prepared myself for a tongue lashing as the two medics checked all my vitals and asked me a ton of questions about my pain and migraine meds, and how much alcohol I drank every day (of course I lied about that). They were incredibly kind.

They seemed concerned about the Imitrex that I'd been using since 1985 for my migraines, and they told me I should talk with my family doctor about referring me to the Ottawa Hospital's Stroke Prevention Clinic (SPC) for a once-a-decade check-up and a meds assessment.

My dear family doctor, Louise Linney, called me as soon as she got the ambulance report. I explained the whole embarrassing mess, and she agreed it would be a good idea to refer me for an assessment at the SPC.

* * *

When I strolled into the Stroke Prevention Clinic, a huge smile grew on the face of the director, Dr. Christine De Meulemeester. She looked vaguely familiar.

"Cathy!" She cheerfully extended her hand to me from behind her desk. "I remember interviewing you for your Botox injections when I worked with Dr. Stys," she confirmed. Pleasantries completed, she sat down to quickly review my intake info. She was all serious now.

"So, you're having a lot of difficulty with chronic pain," she said to herself, then looked up. "And we have to take you off the Imitrex," she said flatly. "It increases your risk of stroke."

My heart sank. Without it, I would not be able to stay in the office four consecutive days a week.

"After we're finished here, I'll bring you over to see Dr. Sitwell, our migraine specialist, and he can give you some alternatives."

"What about cannabis?" (At that time we were both talking about smoking it, unaware that ingestible cannabis oil would later become available. The oil is much safer, since it reaches the bloodstream without damage to the lungs or heart.)

She shook her head. "No. It also increases your risk of stroke." She didn't offer any other explanation. I assumed, like with everything else, research had uncovered new findings.

Dr. Sitwell was very kind, and he gave me a bit of hope.

"There are also other medications you can take every day to help prevent migraines and manage your chronic pain, like pregabalin," he continued. "It was originally developed as an anti-seizure medication to treat epilepsy, but it's been found to have a nice side effect of reducing the frequency and severity of migraines in some people. There are other meds you can try too. You and your family doctor can work together to determine what works best for you."

I nodded and thanked him. I felt heartened that there were

some options open to me, but I was still going to have to take a chunk of time off work until my body felt comfortable enough with the imperative reboot.

* * *

Feeling let down but determined, who should I run into next on the way to Neurology's sixth-floor elevator but dear Dr. Skinner. Even though we hadn't seen each other since 1984, we had learned some amazingly coincidental news about each other over the years.

"Oh, what a nice surprise!" he exclaimed happily. "How are you?"

"Same here! I can't complain. Just finished a check-up for this decade at the Stroke Prevention Clinic."

"That's great," he said, giving me no indication he was in a hurry to move on.

Dr. Skinner was, without a doubt, the kindest and most empathetic physician who treated me after my first stroke in 1984, and with good reason. He too was a parent of an infant girl the same age as our darling baby girl. And as a further crazy coincidence, his daughter ended up in the same Grade 1 class as ours, in a French Catholic school! (Dr. Skinner's wife was a Francophone, just like JP.)

For several years on the occasional weekend, Jean-Pierre drove the two girls back and forth to each other's houses for school projects and playdates, and they remained friends until they changed schools after Grade 6.

"How's your daughter?" I asked. He glowed when I spoke her name.

"Oh, she's great – married and living in Toronto now. And yours?"

"She's so amazing," I gushed. "She's doing a research project on setting up a safe injection site in Victoria at UVic with the Centre for Addictions Research BC (now called the Canadian Institute for Substance Use Research)."

His eyes sparkled. "Wow, that's amazing. I'm so happy she's doing so well."

"You have no idea how much you helped us back then," I told him.

"Well, I might have a bit of an idea. You look like you're doing amazingly well, too."

I nodded, reminded of how grim things were in the beginning, and how he and Dr. Mallya always gave me something positive to hang onto.

"By the way, what's Dr. Mallya doing now?"

"Oh, thank you for asking," he said, becoming serious. "Dr. Mallya went on to become a highly respected neurosurgeon in the U.S., but then he had a couple of really bad heart attacks, and he wasn't able to do surgery anymore."

"Oh, how awful!"

"Yes, it is." Dr. Skinner brought a finger up to his scalp and rubbed it a couple of times, and his sombre expression morphed into surprisingly cheerful bemusement. "But you know what? … I heard he's now leading some sort of … spiritual group," he said, with an embarrassed smile. "I have no idea what it's all about, though."

"You're kidding."

"No, I'm not," he insisted.

"Well, there certainly was a 'presence' about him," I offered, and Dr. Skinner nodded in agreement.

Our exchange reminded me both how far I'd come since 1984, but also how much extra mindfulness I must continually practise just to help rebuild my capacity to interpret the short-circuited loss of sensations that my jumbled brain continues to perceive. Initially, I had almost a complete loss of proprioception, but over years and years, with the screaming "stingies" calmed by time, meds and surgeries, I have found different ways to "perceive" touch. For example, when I've inadvertently put my huge keychain into my right pocket, my right hand can now find the hole, dig in and grasp about to find something pointy like a key digging into a finger that causes discomfort because it's metal, so I know it's the keychain. At first, it would fall to the ground as soon as I lashed it out of my pocket and before I could see how I was holding it. Now, after years of practice, I can "lightly" hang onto it. That's neuroplasticity.

Dr. Skinner and I exchanged pleasant it-was-great-to-see-you-again goodbyes, and as I headed for the parking lot, the more enjoyable memories of the caregivers who helped me thrive reverted to the current most pressing this-is-what-I-gotta-do-now's.

Deep down, I knew my working days were pretty much over. Now that I had to give up Imitrex for migraines, there was no way I'd be able to make it into the office even four days a week, and I would need at least a few weeks to sort things out with new meds.

22

Knowing When It's Over

Jean-Pierre and I threw our family doctor Louise Linney a hard curveball at her next Monday evening clinic, when she opened the door to find us both waiting for her.

"Hey there, what's up?" she asked carefully.

In my impatient, overly direct style when I was stressed, I dove right into the Stroke Prevention Clinic's decree that I must stop taking Imitrex and get on a preventative migraine medication instead, and that I could write a letter from her to my employer explaining that I needed to take a few weeks off to adjust.

"Woah!" poor Louise reacted, completely blindsided. "This was only supposed to be a 15-minute appointment."

"I know, I'm sorry. I just really needed to see you."

"Oh no worries," she said, more calmly, and after a bit more discussion, she agreed it made sense for me to take a few weeks off.

"And I agree with Dr. Sitwell; I think pregabalin would be a good long-term migraine prevention medication for you to try. The only thing is, you cannot drink alcohol on it."

My heart sank. "Okay, that's fine," I lied.

Dr. Linney scheduled another half-hour "talk" appointment for me in two weeks' time, thus initiating the complicated, plodding bureaucratic process of my final descent into early retirement due to disability.

Many doctors want to avoid all the required reports and paperwork related to applying for long-term or permanent disability – or they charge fees for every single document they prepare or sign, making it even more difficult for patients already struggling with disabilities to get the kind of coverage they could be eligible for. I was fortunate that my disabilities, while virtually invisible, were quantifiable by a CT scan proving I had brain damage. Many disability applicants with complex issues, who suffer much more than I have, can fall through the cracks for many reasons. Perhaps they or their caregivers cannot properly explain exactly what's happening to them or the (authoritative or overly self-confident) physician they trust does not have the extended training or unique experience required to make the proper assessment or referral to a specialist who does. Thus, there is always a need for second opinions. They never hurt.

When I was first told that I must forever abstain from the demon Johnnie Walker and Chardonnay, JP promptly decided to stop drinking alcohol and smoking marijuana to make it easier on me. Right away, he stopped cold.

I, however, struggled to give up alcohol for another year. I still loved the intoxicating scents, holding the stem and sipping from my giant glass (or two) of delectable wine with dinner, along with frozen margaritas on the deck, especially when friends came over, and I kept insisting my occasional indulgence wasn't a big deal

Until our daughter came home from university for a visit.

After finishing dessert from the lovely dinner she and Poppa Hen prepared, I heard her set down her spoon. Then she frankly told me that I was nearly comatose, and that I had to stop drinking. There is nothing worse than having your child tell you they are disappointed in you. And nothing more motivating.

"You're right. I'm so sorry, honey," I mumbled in shame, my voice tiny. "I promise, I'll stop."

And I did.

It took my daughter's concern for me to make me finally accept how much they'd both supported me, and how much I needed their tough love to avoid falling down a black hole I would never climb back up from.

And then, there was another ultimatum a few years later, when she finally convinced me to get hearing aids.

After breakfast, near the end of our first glorious Mom-Daughter all-inclusive, week-long winter getaway to Jamaica, she carefully laid down her cutlery again and said that she would not go on another trip with me unless I got hearing aids, because every time she or a server or anyone else said anything, I would ask them to repeat themselves, and it was extremely annoying.

I didn't argue with her. I had tried hearing aids about 10 years previously, but gave up on them because the technology didn't seem to be advanced enough to help. Only three days after we returned to our land of ice and snow, I scurried to Costco and got myself one of the first types of hearing aids that synced with an iPhone so that I could listen to music while walking, as well as converse without having to hold the phone to my ear. I just love it, and I love my daughter even more for knowing how to encourage me.

To this day, I remain on pregabalin, and JP and I enjoy making delicious non-alcoholic beverages. My current favourite is a tall icy mixture of sparkling mineral water, a small swoosh of unsweetened cranberry and mango juices, a splash of lime, and a sprig of fresh mint.

When JP and I went to Spain in 2014, non-alcoholic cerveza was available at every beach bar and bistro, all the time – even a de-alcoholized Stella Artois!

There's a much wider variety of alcohol-free products available in Canada now than there was back in 2007. We are particularly fond of Corona Sunbrew 0.0% alcohol beer and VI-NO-ZE-RO, a German white available only across the river in "la belle province de Québec," particularly beer and spritzer-type concoctions. Atypique, another company from Quebec, makes "mocktails" that are superb, especially their killer "gin" and tonic. And now there's even de-alcoholized Tanqueray gin in North America! Gotta try it!

* * *

Going on long-term disability is complicated and stressful, even for someone like me, who has worked and lived in bureaucracy. I was lucky to have quantifiable neurological disabilities supported by brain scans, an exceptional family doctor and an employer who continued to support me from day one. Many others with more nebulous conditions, like fibromyalgia, chronic fatigue syndrome, sudden severe allergies, autoimmune disorders and scores of other hard-to-document conditions, often require independent assessments from doctors unfamiliar with the complexities of the applicant's issues. Also, by the time that person reaches the point where they can no longer cope, it becomes harder and harder to jump through all the hoops to complete the required paperwork within the prescribed time periods. And even then, after all the medical appointments, examinations and certified documentation, the financial support they very well should be entitled to can be refused. Perhaps they or their caregiver doesn't know how to explain the issues, symptoms and limitations in a way that fits the accepted medical definitions of "disability."

Before I first went on long-term disability in 2007, I had to use up all my vacation leave, then all my sick leave, (which didn't matter since I was already in arrears), and then go on leave without pay for several months before the reduced payments kicked in. How can a person with disabilities who lives alone or without financial stability manage to do this?

In August 2023, *The Globe and Mail* reported that 6.2 million Canadians – that's one in five – live with a physical, developmental or psychiatric disability. Forty per cent of Canadians living in poverty have a disability.

Back to 2007, I was visited at home by Anne Gourlay, a rehabilitation consultant from Sun Life. We chatted for two hours; it was exhausting, and she took copious notes, while also offering me microwavable heating pads and for the tub, a grab bar, bathtub chair and removable showerhead to make my life easier. Extremely accommodating.

"I understand that your employer is working out a part-time assignment for you in collaboration with your family doctor that would involve working from home?"

"Yes, that's my understanding."

"Perfect."

She stood up and shook my hand. "It's been a pleasure meeting you, Cathy, and I'll enjoy working with you to help you to reintegrate back to work."

I falsely smiled bravely, even though I already knew it was over.

* * *

We were now playing the workplace wage-replacement, disability-insurance game. The process is plagued with a plethora of ambiguous rules that sometimes seem contradictory, and every bureaucrat and medical expert from the Department of Justice, Sun Life and ultimately, Health Canada and the Canada Revenue Agency would need their own form of data and documentation to justify my increasing inability to perform, even under the most accommodating circumstances by the employer.

But wow, the Department of Justice went beyond my wildest dreams in their efforts to accommodate every last ounce of my off-kilter brain power. Under the direction of continuous correspondence with my amazing physician, Dr. Linney, (mostly drafted by me and signed by her), and Sun Life's Rehabilitation officer,

Justice made the tough road as pleasant as possible for me, right to the very end, and I'm forever grateful.

The approval process for going on work replacement wages, long-term disability and ultimately, a federal disability pension is often much, much harder than what I experienced. I was extremely fortunate in that my issue; stroke, or cerebral vascular accident, fit a medically cut and dried definition of disability, and all the players always found a way to agree with each other. But I still had to play the game by the rules, and even for me, it was no picnic.

While many physicians also charge fees for every single document, letter or form they are required to produce or sign, Dr. Linney never charged me a cent, and she was always quick to refer me to an expert whenever a new health issue popped up.

Almost everything costs more when you have disabilities. Everything you might need to do things "differently" can require some sort of adaptive technology or special equipment. Like a left-foot gas pedal. But if you or your healthcare workers are not attuned to the latest innovations, you may miss out on key opportunities for recovery or maintaining yourself.

There are the financial advisors and companies that exist to help people with disabilities claim income tax benefits and refunds, sometimes over periods of decades that they had no idea they were eligible for. All for a fee, of course, along with supporting medical documentation; and more fees …

However, I was blessed that my dear friend, Vera Adamovich, helped me navigate the miasma of our more complex taxation reporting. Vera was a systems analyst who I worked with at EDC and was one of the few individuals I'd kept in touch with after my first stroke. We lost contact for several years after I had my second one, and during this time she became a certified financial planner and set up her own business, currently known as Create Wealth Management.

We eventually reconnected, and now Vera's firm handles all of our financial needs with unwavering kindness and efficiency. She is the one who initially pointed out my entitlement to over $12K of unclaimed federal income tax refunds. As well, she let me know that prescribed mobility aids such as a left-foot gas pedal can be claimed as medical expenses on income tax returns. She was also instrumental in helping me manage my father's descent into dementia and protected me from fraud in settling his estate after his passing in July 2019.

What a guardian angel!

No wonder that so many Canadians with disabilities can do nothing but wallow in poverty and die alone if they don't have the knowledge, support from family and friends, or the mental or physical stamina to cope with all the added burdens of being their own best advocate.

* * *

For my final three-month rehabilitation assignment, I worked three half-days a week – Monday and Friday mornings at home, with only Wednesday mornings at the office downtown. My workspace was in the windowless basement inside the stately Justice library – very quiet, and surprisingly pleasant …

Again, the Department of Justice went to extraordinary lengths to accommodate me in my home office, setting up my ergonomically adjusted chair and a computer interface with extra special access to JUSnet, the employees-only intranet site. I was one of the first few Justice employees to be granted this "for-use-on-Justice-locations-only" exemption, and I was sternly cautioned not to allow anyone else access to this confidential website.

While I enjoyed my final assignment and felt I was still contributing to the well-being of the department, my migraines were still frequent and debilitating, even on the near-maximum, four-times-a-day doses of pregabalin, and often, I couldn't work for even the allotted three mornings per week. The project I was engaged in was running behind schedule. I was losing the battle.

Still, I'll never forget the surprise phone call I received one Wednesday morning while I was working in the Justice library, a few weeks before the completion date of my assignment.

"Hi Cathy, it's Gord Boyle, Manager of Disability Services from Sun Life's head office in Montreal." I had spoken with Gord once before and had previously received a few letters from him on administrative details, so he was not unknown to me.

"I've gone over your file," he began, "And it's clear that you are having a hard time. I just wanted to let you know that if you agree, I am going to recommend you stop working and receive wage replacement benefits till age 65."

Wow. It was all over. Just like that.

I had mixed feelings. First, huge relief, but at the same time, overwhelming guilt about bailing on the project before it was completed.

Regardless, I prepared a letter for Dr. Linney in the required "bureau-speak" to officially agree with everyone that my career was over.

Above all, I am grateful that I helped pay off our mortgage and enabled our daughter to go to her chosen universities without being saddled with heavy post-grad student debt.

* * *

A couple of weeks after the end of my fulfilling career of more than a decade at Justice, I got a call from Virginia McRae, my former ADM of the Management Sector, and now a Professor of Law at the University of Ottawa.

"We're having a town hall meeting for the Management Sector to encourage employees to self-identify if they have disability issues," she began. "We've developed a form that people can complete to help their supervisors out, and I'd be delighted if you would come and talk to us for a few minutes about your self-identification experience with us at Justice."

"Really?"

"Yes, and you won't be the only speaker. I've also asked Michel Francoeur to join us to tell his own story."

Michel Francoeur? That totally hot, bald lawyer who all the women go gaga over? He has a disability?

"Oh, thank you for asking me, Virginia. It would be an honour."

* * *

I had become fairly well-known across the Department as the editor of *inter pares* and *JustInfo,* particularly after I obtained permission to rerun a piece written by my husband about me entitled

"Comfortably Numb," which appeared in *Ottawa City Woman* magazine in September 2004.

The feedback from that Friday's *JustInfo* was phenomenal. When I returned to the office on Tuesday, I was shocked to find more than 100 laudatory emails in my inbox, many from people I'd never had the pleasure of meeting. Even Deputy Attorney General Daniel Bellemare, who had previously been livid over my sloppy editing procedure of the article on his epic visit with Nelson Mandella, expressed glowing admiration. My Associate Director-General of Communications, Jean Valin, also stopped me in the hallway as I returned from one of my rare, always joyous lunch-hour treks up Parliament Hill, past the Chateau Laurier lookout and through to the magnificent grounds of Major's Hill Park.

"Thanks so much for sharing that great piece your husband wrote," he said. "I had absolutely no idea of what you're dealing with."

* * *

Still, I was petrified when Virginia called me to the microphone at the town hall meeting. Michel Francoeur noticed my hands were trembling.

"You'll do fine," he whispered, as I carefully stepped up to the mike.

How ironic it was that I would be so spooked. Granted, it was my first time giving a speech, even though I had written a few for officials at Secretary of State and Export Development Corporation. When I was just a pup in marketing at EDC, I'd been tasked with "speech coaching" a few pious executives while coordinating logistics for the corporation's national seminar programs. (When coaching the higher-ups, it was understood that only basic encouragement was tolerated, like "make sure your microphone is properly positioned before speaking, maintain eye contact with your audience, try to avoid fidgeting, reading your words, or speaking too quickly.")

Many brilliant people are hopeless as public speakers.

But it wasn't until it was my turn to officially open my mouth that I understood why many people are more afraid of public speaking than death.

Once I got started though, I was fine. I explained my various altered states, and that because they were invisible, for the most part, I had no choice but to inform management up front if I ever wanted to work again. To get the job, I had to first promote my abilities, of course, but since my issues (particularly in a communications environment) required quite a major accommodation back then, (as in working a four-day week instead of five), my employer had to know the "whats" and "hows" before they could be in a position to collaborate.

In my presentation, I discussed how having a disability often feels embarrassing or demeaning because others cannot help but make instant judgements about your mental competence the moment they see you. It's also your legal right to keep your health issues confidential. But whether a disability is visible or invisible, an individual's chances of surviving in the workforce require, at the very least, an honest conversation about it with your employer, along with medical documentation supporting your situation. Your boss needs to know from a certified professional what kinds of circumstances aggravate your issues and whether you need any specific kind of accommodation, however insignificant or frivolous it might seem to them.

(I did not talk about this in my presentation, but even after identifying yourself as a person with disabilities, you can still face resentment from a supervisor or a colleague who may perceive you to be "lazy," "entitled" or "unsuitable for promotion." This actually happened to me once at Justice. It was very personal and nasty, and it nearly broke me. I don't want to go into specifics, but once senior management learned about the situation, and because I had self-identified, the problem was quickly put to rest.)

I continued to discuss other examples of accommodation issues in the workplace – perhaps someone with epilepsy might need lower lighting to help reduce the risk of them having a seizure. Someone else can go into anaphylactic shock just from the smell of something they are allergic to, and it's not only peanut butter. It could be anything: shellfish, jalapeno peppers, fruit, perfumes or intimate products. No two people react the same way to everything.

Often the accommodation required is not terribly complicated, and if you already know exactly what you need to optimize your performance, all the better. Other times, even a "simple" accommodation effort can result in failure after failure. Maybe a technician didn't interpret the need exactly the same way as the person who expressed it; a specialist recommended something that was not quite right; or maybe the issue wasn't initially explained the right way. Or perhaps, by the time the accommodation was finally made, the employee deteriorated further. Accommodation in the workplace can be a nightmare and can sometimes be so difficult or costly that it scares off prospective employers.

Things can often get messy when someone returns to work after some sort of setback. Since the person often looks the same as before, everyone thinks they're just like they used to be, but they're not. They come back too soon and can't cope. Maybe they need some sort of accommodation but don't even realize it. Perhaps they are too proud or too scared to even ask. Or they don't bother following up with their doctor. Or the doctor insists there shouldn't be an issue. And that's why the immediate members of your team should also know if your issues change, even if no accommodation is required.

After I finished thanking the department for helping me achieve what I often feared was an impossible dream, the large group sustained several seconds of spirited applause. Michel Francoeur grinned and gave me a thumbs up as I successfully made it back to my chair without tripping on the mat. Then Virginia introduced Michel, and he strode confidently to the mike.

When he opened his mouth, it curled sideways, and he began to speak in loud, choppy, almost unintelligible forced rushes. It was all I could do to keep my own mouth from dropping open in disbelief.

Michel told us he just woke up one morning and his ability to speak had become rudely distorted. I was so discombobulated that I couldn't absorb all his details, but it was a neurological issue. The good news is that this vibrant man was able to remain at Justice as a general counsel in public law.

I feel so blessed to have worked with such a committed group of forward-thinking individuals who do their best to create and amend our country's laws to reflect the governing political party's ideals for the security and well-being of all Canadians, notwithstanding all our ongoing inequities, hidden and overt racism, and particularly, but not exclusively, our treatment of Indigenous peoples and other minorities. Supremely difficult tasks, indeed. But never doubt the efforts of the public servants at Canada's Department of Justice – their efforts are pure gold.

My previous struggles to be physically present in the office are almost a non-issue for employees nowadays, with remote work from home becoming the new normal out of necessity, to protect workers and our global economies during the COVID-19 pandemic. Not to ignore the unbearable social pressures this placed on families with two breadwinners and children forced to stay home from school and quarantine together, the pandemic blew open the need for flexibility in the workplace and provided more freedoms at work for those with personal issues.

Round III

23

Getting Back My Groove with Neurophysio and Yoga

Many of us may know of someone who becomes ill as soon as they take time off work, or even worse, passes away soon after retirement. Maybe it's the only time they've ever allowed themselves to relax, and once they do, they discover they've got more health problems that they didn't have time to notice or confront.

That pretty much describes me.

The paperwork that started the transition from me receiving the long-term disability work replacement benefit to my official retirement due to disability dragged on until 2013. That's right – four years of bureaucratic foot-dragging, and my case was cut and dried. I shudder to think how much more difficult this would be for someone who does not have all their faculties, stamina or support from others to weather this sort of ongoing financial stress.

That in itself is debilitating.

In 2009, I was back in the nice warm aquafit pool with Pat, Gail and Elaine on Tuesday and Thursday mornings, and trying to go for walks every day, even if only for 10 or 15 minutes. In those days, sitting down at bus stop benches was a regular component of the routes I chose. As I've described, I used these opportunities to rest, breathe and reorient my posture by balancing my sitz bones and then mindfully placing both feet flat and equidistantly apart, before rising back to a standing position. Still, my whole world seemed to centre on managing my worsening chronic pain and fatigue.

I told Dr. Linney that I was desperate for more relief.

"Well, I can only suggest two options," she told me. She knew I was desperate. "Morphine, which is very hard on your system, or cannabis, which is still illegal, so you'd have to acquire it through your own sources…"

"But with weed, you'd have no idea of the consistency in potency or quality, right?"

She nodded. "Yes. Exactly."

"Okay then, put me on morphine," I muttered, knowing that this was a major step downhill.

The morphine helped a great deal at first, but eventually made me feel like a brain-dead zombie. Dr. Linney wasn't kidding when she said it is hard on your system. It shuts everything down.

Every morning, the first priority and biggest bane of my existence turned into going for a dump in the morning.

My search for relief from chronic constipation seemed

never-ending. Life couldn't start till I had that blasted poo. I had been swallowing sickening orange globs of Metamucil on a regular basis since my early twenties, but now it wasn't doing squat.

The only thing at that point that made the biggest difference was walking.

And so walking became my religion.

I walked and walked and walked. As much as I could.

Until my right heel started to get so sore I could barely keep weight on it.

The Ottawa Hospital's Rehabilitation Centre was still giving me regular foot care, and when I mentioned my sore heel to managing chiropodist Ruth Thompson, the first thing she said was, "You need new shoes."

She was right. My beloved supportive hipster shoes had gone soft around the ankles, and the soles were unevenly worn down.

Ruth had one of her students cover my entire heel with white adhesive skin tape. "You should keep your ankle taped all the time, even when you go in the pool," she told me. "And then you can reapply it afterwards when you're dried off and getting dressed.

"Hmm, that'll be so much fun," I said gloomily.

"I'm also going to refer you to a physiatrist for a diagnosis," Ruth told me. "Hopefully that won't take too long."

Physical Medicine and Rehabilitation expert Dr. Meenaxi Acharya was quick to tell me it was plantar fasciitis that was causing my heel pain. The tissue that connects the heel to the toe through the arch often shrinks or becomes inflamed as we age, and one of the best ways to relieve the pain is to stretch that tissue, by walking.

However, a spastically paralyzed foot does not lend itself to self-directed stretching. Also, the tendons that were Zorro-lengthened and shifted around during my foot reconstruction to pull the gone-wonky appendage into a flatter, more walkable position had been securely wound together into a round lump the size of a penny, high inside my arch.

However, my right foot and ankle were surprisingly flexible when manipulated with massage, physiotherapy or my own hands, and there were several exercises I could do myself – like positioning a small, hard Theraball on top of a cushion to help keep the foot stable on top of it, and then pressing down as hard as I could tolerate in different areas under the arch for at least two minutes. It remains a chronic condition that must be managed, and it's another reason why I have grown to love walking so much.

Move it or lose it.

And Theraballs. These small, hard, rubbery exercise balls are great for releasing kinks and knots almost anywhere, with a bit of consistent pressure for a few minutes.

"I also want the Rehab Centre to make you some custom orthotic inserts," Dr. Acharya continued. "And you need to see a neurological physiotherapist. The front desk at the main entrance can provide you with a list of neurological physiotherapists in private practice."

Dr. Acharya was a cheerful woman with light chocolate skin, intensely happy eyes and long, black hair. She was always a wonderful listener with a kind, engaging aura who always tried to give positive, practical suggestions. She was also an assistant professor of Physical Medicine and Rehabilitation at the University of Ottawa. Over the years she gave me Botox injections at Elisabeth Bruyère Continuing Care hospital and all sorts of valuable advice whenever I was referred back to her for follow-up. This busy rehabilitation specialist was also a consultant to the Rehab Centre and other Ottawa hospitals. I had hoped that should I ever again require her expertise, she would be, at the very least, in well-deserved semi-retirement.

But sadly, she passed away on April 23, 2023. Life can be so unfair for some.

* * *

I first met my new neurological physiotherapist, Lucie Hemstead, at M.A.P. Physiotherapy in 2011. This clinic treats complex cases in pediatric, perinatal, orthopedic and neurological physiotherapy. To this day, Lucie remains my for-life physiotherapist.

She worked on the neurological ward of Windsor Regional Hospital for four years, and now runs her own practice from her lovely, private home studio. I still drive 40 kilometres across town from Orléans to see her regularly every few weeks, or sometimes more often, if needed. Lucie knows every evolving quirk in my body better than anyone, and she seldom fails to tune up the most demanding pains of the month as if she's keeping her vintage car humming along.

And how does she do it?

With a combination of different tools – all with the goal of finding balance. Alignment, awareness and breathing are the main elements. Finding and creating a stable base of support in all postures ideally allows the best movement control. The basis of her analysis is often the Bobath concept, which is often used for stroke patients and children with cerebral palsy, and involves neurological assessment, understanding motor control and promoting motor learning to help patients better understand what they're dealing with. She often uses other techniques as well, such as myofascial release and facilitation of normal movements to achieve these goals.

Ever pull away the elastic white tissue under the skin of a chicken breast? That's fascia. Fascia is connective tissue, and it's everywhere in the human body. It holds organs, muscles, blood vessels and nerve fibres in place, connecting all of our systems. Fascia can get twisted and seize up, just like muscles. And when there's a kink in the fascia somewhere, whatever's connected to it may not move the way it should anymore. When stroke and other neurological issues, such as muscular dystrophy, cause high spasticity – which in turn can cause muscles to atrophy and shrink over time – this shrinkage puts chronic stress on the fascia surrounding the muscle, and causes pain. Therefore, sometimes before you can relieve a tight muscle, you must first release the fascia.

Lucie's training in myofascial release along with neurological movement analysis leads to improved functioning of a patient. The fascia is detected, through her fingertips, where the fascia is kinked up, and through continuous and (usually) gentle pressure, the stressed fascia can be released so that pain is reduced, and subsequently, the muscle can move more freely, allowing more access to muscle and movement control.

The greater portion of my first hour-long appointment with

Lucie was of course to assess my overall condition, in addition to my most recently diagnosed symptoms of plantar fasciitis. It had been close to a decade since I'd had any physiotherapy, and since 1990, it was always with an orthopedic physiotherapist, someone who nearly always provided repetitive exercise treatment to muscles, tendons and bones. None of these treatments ever seemed very effective for me.

I also had no idea how twisted up my muscles had become, only that I hurt all over, all the time. Even my stronger left side was cranky after years and years of bearing the brunt of steadying my weaker side. Morphine was the most recent addition to my growing list of painkillers, but it was shutting my body down and numbing my brain along with it.

Bowel movements were excruciating, exhausting and too few and far between. Back then, my day could not start until I'd had my morning BM. All these morbidly intimate details were provided to Lucie, and after about a half hour of questions, her physical fact-finding mission began.

"We'll get you all sorted out," she said calmly.

Really? That's the first time anyone's actually told me that ...

"Okay, I'm just going to slowly move different parts of your body to check your range of motion and your sensitivities, and I want you to tell me as soon as it gets too uncomfortable. I'm going to start with your right shoulder."

"Okay ... ARGHH! F**K!"

I felt so embarrassed crying out like that. Lucie had barely touched me, and her face froze in surprise when I yelped. She must have wondered if my strokes had left me aphasic and prone to outbursts of profanity.

"So sorry! I don't usually swear like that."

"Oh, no worries," she said softly. "You know, it's a good thing you got here when you did. Your shoulder's almost frozen."

I couldn't believe it. "Really?" She nodded, with a sweet smile. "We can fix it."

Lucie Hemstead gave me the knowledge and power to heal myself, and the confidence to do it.

One of the first things she told me to do every day was to "go lightly." Imagine my affected arm and leg are weightless. Don't force the movement; let the movement come, as if you're a ballet dancer. I still practise this when I bend down to unload the dishwasher and reach up to the cupboards holding plates and cups. Hurry too much, and I'll go all jerky and spastic.

Slow is good. So very good.

At first I had doubts that she could "fix me up," and I'd say it took a good year of weekly visits before I realized I was walking better and faster than ever. Now I can even keep up with Jean-Pierre (or, on occasion, make him keep up with me). Mind you, he has slowed down with his own issues. But for the first time since 1984, we could hold hands while walking in sync with each other. Such a romantic gift!

With my new-found increased flexibility, I found the courage to get more into yoga. I had taken my first kundalini yoga class at Colonel By High School after my first stroke. The emphasis in this yoga class was on breathing and meditation while lying on the floor, which suited me perfectly. I felt shy and embarrassed not being able to do the poses the same way as everyone else, and I did not dare do any practice at home, as I feared ridicule from my still-stuck-on-aerobic-exercise husband, as in "What-the-f***are you doing?"

After the second stroke, leaving home to participate in a yoga class was next to impossible. By the time I got into my attire, gathered the yoga mat and drove to class, I was already exhausted. A few yoga instructors even gave me seriously negative attitude when I had to insist to them that I could not go barefoot because one foot was numb and seized-up, and I needed to wear non-slip aqua shoes just to keep my balance. Again, invisible disabilities can often lead to misconceptions, even among those who consider themselves to espouse "universal love."

So I gave up on yoga then, too. Until 2010.

I found a book in the library entitled *Boomer Yoga: Energizing the Years Ahead for Men and Women,* by Beryl Bender Birch. Her approach to adapting a pose to suit your own physicality resonated with me. I decided I needed to figure out how to set up my own yoga practice at home because of the seizing fibromyalgia-like pain that I needed to deal with as soon as I opened my eyes every morning, just to get my old dented jalopy of a body putt-putting, and to hell with what my poses looked like or how I looked doing it.

Around the same time as I was in yoga research mode, I spotted a Groupon ad I couldn't refuse.

"Live Your Yoga" was offering eight one-hour sessions for $20 per session, in your own home, tailored to your own specific needs, from a certified yogini (a female master of yoga). I leapt at the opportunity.

Not long after, my new yoga experiment was set to begin. Monica Chappell rang my doorbell at exactly 7 p.m. She was a tall, quietly peaceful beauty. Her long, wavy dark hair fell past her shoulders to her long, lithe arms and legs, and she carried a small ghetto blaster and a shoulder bag with her yoga mat and other essentials.

We did our sessions every Wednesday night in the darkened living room, with the coffee table pushed aside and Monica's gentle new-age music providing a calming balm. She subscribed to the teachings of yogi Don Stapleton, Ph.D., author of another fabulous reference book entitled, *Self-Awakening Yoga: The Expansion of Consciousness through the Body's Own Wisdom*. He explains how you can develop an intuitive way of moving based on what your body needs. I devoured this book; it spoke to me.

Together, Monica and I figured out that for starters, what I needed most was to improve my breathing. I would lie on the floor, relax my anxious mind and do gentle stretching from that position. I would then concentrate my breath towards the area being stretched, gradually move to a sitting position, and continue to hold other extremely simple positions and relax into them.

"I am learning a lot from you about the importance of stilling the mind," she told me. "I'm going to pass this on to my own mother. She has fibromyalgia, and she's really enjoying getting into yoga now too."

After the initial eight $20 Groupon sessions, Monica offered to continue weekly visits at the same philanthropic price, and we enjoyed another month together. Then she decided to go work on an organic farm in Metcalfe, Ontario.

On the day of our last session, I opened the front door to find her grinning from ear to ear, her head shaved completely bald.

"I donated my hair to cancer," she said proudly.

Monica taught me the power of loving my physical body and nurturing it. She was truly an angel sent to me from out of the blue; all I did was accept her call.

24

Pelvic Physio, Massage Therapy and Naturopathy

Around the same time, I began to experience constant bladder leakage when I laughed, along with urinary tract infections that stung when I peed, as well as painful sex and continued horrendous constipation.

"I learned recently there's a physiotherapist close by who specializes in women with pelvic issues," Dr. Linney said. "A few of my patients have had great success with her."

My neuro physio Lucie Hemstead had already given me a heads-up about what pelvic physiotherapists do. "An amazing colleague of mine, Andrea Plitz, does pelvic physiotherapy," she had explained. "She actually inserts her gloved fingers into your vagina to assess scar tissue, myofascial issues and other stress that may exist, and she can actually treat those issues that connect with the pelvis internally. It's something I'd actually like to learn to do one day. It's just an awesome way to treat women because we can develop all sorts of problems down there."

First, I went to the pelvic physiotherapist recommended by my family doctor. From this professional, I learned that there are four stages of pelvic prolapse; stages I and II are treatable with physiotherapy, while stages III and IV require surgical intervention.

When she finished the internal examination, she looked up at me, her face grave.

"I'm so sorry, Cathy," she pronounced. "You have stage III pelvic prolapse. I can offer you biofeedback treatment combined with exercises that may provide some relief, but you will probably require surgery."

Okay, this was discouraging news, but still, I purchased the biofeedback equipment out of pocket for a couple hundred bucks and returned to see her once a week for about a month.

She inserted the metal whatchamacallit into my vagina, which connected to a computer.

"Now, at random intervals," she explained, "the computer will tell you to "contract," and your internal device will vibrate. Every time this occurs, pull your vagina up as high as you can towards your pelvic floor, and then release it. Sometimes the intervals between the commands will be quite brief, so you'll have to pull and let go very quickly, okay?"

"All right, let's do this," I said, hoping that biofeedback was going to be at least as fun as going on a tea-cup ride at a country fair.

But it wasn't.

I still have vivid memories of this therapist glowering over me, and applying hard, burning, two-fingered slaps on my affected side with every CONTRACT command I missed or fell behind at, as if that was going to help stimulate my vagina to become more punctual.

"Please, stop slapping my right leg," I implored, on several occasions. "It just increases my spasticity and makes it even harder for me to make isolated movements."

She just didn't get it, though. The biofeedback indeed gave me some increased awareness of my numbed and weakened pelvic areas, but it was the only pelvic treatment therapy she provided, and for me, it was extremely unpleasant.

I did relay her stage III diagnosis to my family doctor, who in turn referred me to Dr. Kevin Baker, a urogynecological surgeon, for a second opinion. In the meantime, I switched pelvic physio-therapists, and went to see Lucie Hemstead's colleague, Andrea Plitz.

Andrea was tiny and pretty, with almost waist-length, light brown hair and looked like she might still get carded at a bar. She was calm, gentle, and oh, so gifted. A genius.

While she conducted the internal exploration, she asked me to let her know at any time if I experienced pain or discomfort, and she would adapt (or scale down) whatever she was doing.

"How's that?"

"Ooohh! Oh, okay, that feels a lot better now." Almost instantly, I could feel some form of release.

"Good." Andrea explained that she would be giving me a few more vaginal treatments to release scar tissue and twisted fascia.

"What about biofeedback?" I asked.

"No, I don't use that," she said. "It's only one form of treatment, and it has its limitations."

When she finished the combined examination/treatment, she smiled and said "I would rate your prolapse at stage II." (And so did Dr. Baker, a bit later.)

"Oh good, so you don't think I'll need surgery then."

"No, no," she assured me. "You'll be fine with the treatment and exercises I'll give you. I should also mention that you have a rectocele."

"Yes," I said, "I learned that when I had my hemorrhoidectomy."

A rectocele is another form of pelvic prolapse where the rectum pushes against the vagina, making it bulge. This can result in a feeling of bloating, painful sex, constipation and even obstructive defecation. Andi showed me how and where to manipulate my fingers to help facilitate the pooping process.

"I'd also recommend you get a squatty potty," she said. It's a raised shelf that goes around the toilet – you can put your feet on it, to get more into a squatting position. That's how early humans used to do it. Much more efficient, and it puts less strain on the pelvis."

Andrea, also a newly-minted yoga instructor, showed me appropriately adapted yoga exercises and even emailed me photos with detailed descriptions of the appropriate positions for me to use. It was almost magical the way she combined several disciplines to treat complex sources of pain in addition to my pelvic issues. Sometimes it seemed like she barely touched me.

I saw Andi on a regular basis for a good four months, and then from time to time after that. The internal therapy was required for only a few sessions; then it became Andi's own expert hybrid physiotherapy and yogic therapy methods that helped strengthen and relax my insides.

Andi suggested I hook up with Jennifer Spak, a multi-talented registered massage therapist and osteopath. One of her many specialties is helping infants who have problems breastfeeding to improve their suckling skills; yet, she was not a massage therapist you'd go to for a relaxing Swedish massage.

Jennifer Spak taught me how to massage my colon several times a day to stimulate it and improve my digestion. She also had me purchase a medium-sized, soft air-filled plastic ball at the dollar store to place at various points underneath my sensitive tummy when I lay on the floor face-down to do my own myofascial release. I was starting to realize how important simple "props" can be in order to "heal thyself."

Jennifer also showed Jean-Pierre how to apply kinesiology tape to my cranky right shoulder before we left for a three-week trip to Spain. Kinesiology tape has been shown to help fatigued muscles perform better, and a study in 2017 indicated that it can help stroke patients improve the way they walk. Physical therapists think it may be because experiencing the strange sensation of tape placed over an affected muscle can remind you or make you more aware of how you're moving. That's probably why Dr. Acharya once suggested I could try wrapping my sensory-affected knee with Saran Wrap, to remind my leg that it can bend if I consciously try to make it do so while I walk.

Back to kinesiology tape – it has a wide range of uses, but there are also some serious contraindications; so it's important to consult a medical professional before you start wrapping yourself up with anything.

Jen also gave me some useful tips for managing tinnitus (sometimes constant, and more-or-less incurable ringing) in my right ear at bedtime. But the most amazing thing she did was refer me to naturopathic doctor Sarah Vadeboncoeur.

The rough translation for Sarah's last name is "to go through life with a good heart," and she embodies this dedication in everything she does.

Sarah helped cure me of my chronic constipation. And how, you might ask?

By having me drink a cup of warm water with a splash of lemon juice every morning and taking magnesium glycinate in the morning and at bedtime.

Magnesium is one of the most important minerals for human health and supports more than 300 functions in our bodies. But most of us are deficient in it. Why? Because most of the foods that used to be considered the most plentiful in magnesium, like fruit and vegetables, no longer contain this important mineral because our soils have been over-farmed, year after year, with acres and acres of massive one-type-only crops. They have also been over-sprayed with harmful chemicals, depleting the nutritional value of everything grown on them, and therefore, everything we eat.

This has also encouraged me to eat more organic foods, which is again, more costly.

Stress also depletes the magnesium in your body, so if you struggle with any kind of chronic health issue, you probably need extra magnesium. It can also be helpful for chronic pain.

But again, ALWAYS check with a healthcare professional you trust before trying any new therapy of any kind.

25

Kicking Morphine with the Fabulous Five and Neuroplasticity

Around Christmas 2015, I learned that medical marijuana was about to be decriminalized, and medical cannabis clinics were starting to open up across Canada to legally prescribe it. From my alcohol-with-a-few-tokes-of-cannabis days at the end of my career, I had already blissfully experienced how well cannabis calmed my chronic burning and high spasticity, and I was further heartened to learn that cannabis had been scientifically proven to reduce spasticity, as well as the severity and frequency of epileptic seizures. (I was already taking pregabalin, a drug originally developed to treat epilepsy, which helps prevent and lessen the severity of my migraine headaches). It was also reassuring that I could obtain cannabis from a credible source, assuring purity, consistent THC/CBD ratios and strength of the product, and that effectiveness dosages would remain consistent.

Dr. Linney willingly referred me to Canadian Cannabis Clinics in January 2016. After a urine test and quick checkup from a staff doctor, I was directed to another private room for my first Skype appointment with a doctor from Kingston, Ontario. She agreed that I was an excellent candidate for cannabis therapy, and we agreed on a THC/CBD ratio that we thought would suit me. We also agreed that Tweed, a local supplier who had recently taken over the old Hershey Chocolate factory in Smiths Falls, Ontario, would be a good supplier.

However, when we got to the form of cannabis I would be using, she threw me for a loop.

"I want you to use cannabis butter," she told me.

"Butter?"

I knew that smoking weed was contraindicated for many of the same reasons as tobacco, but I had no idea what other forms were available in Canada. I hoped that I could use pills, or even better, a spray.

Back in 2015, when we were in Granada, Spain, enjoying a magical breakfast near the open-air agora nestled inside the walls of our 800-year-old hotel, I will never forget the friendly, congenial couple about our age, seated within chatting distance. They were from San Francisco. It was the first state in the U.S. to decriminalize marijuana.

The woman mentioned she had noticed me sitting in the agora the day before, carefully rationing my big bag of beloved drugs into the chambers of my weekly plastic pill box. As the four of us got to chatting, we discovered that we all dealt with serious health issues, and how that made us even more grateful to be in this breathtaking village – with its white walled architecture, sprinkled with deep red geraniums and framed by the dark green spires of Cypress trees and the white-capped Sierra Nevada mountain range – despite our limitations.

Then the gentleman took a discreet little canister out of his shirt pocket and popped a long spray of cannabis oil under his tongue.

"I wouldn't be here without this," he declared. "It's so quick and effective."

Actually, this man was extremely lucky he wasn't discovered going through customs and arrested for bringing his weed spray across international borders. Police dogs trained to detect the campy scent are often dispatched to roam and sniff out every bag and every passenger waiting in line to check in on international flights. To this day, it remains a grave offence to transport any form of cannabis almost everywhere in the world (except maybe Uruguay, last time I checked).

Anyway, back to the limited approved selection of cannabis products in Canada at that time … my new weed doc told me there was a recipe in the welcome folder I'd been given. "You basically have to bake your cannabis in the oven at a specific temperature, then simmer it in oil and drain it."

Ewww! I don't want our house to smell like a grow-op!

Not only that, but JP had enough hassles being our house chef and cleaner, and with my disabilities, I just didn't want to get into cooking my own oil – it would be, again, too difficult to ensure consistent dosage, and with my affected hand, too dangerous to handle.

After meeting with Brad Pichette, my cannabis counsellor who subsequently prepared all the necessary paperwork for me to sign, I went home, feeling quite distressed. Weren't there any suppliers in Canada offering pre-made cannabis oil?

I went online and checked out Tweed's website. At that time, they did not offer cannabis oil. Eventually I discovered that CanniMed, a company in Saskatchewan and actually the first legal cannabis producer in Canada, offered oil in the THC/CBD ratio recommended for me. It was expensive: over $100 for a bottle that would last about a month, but I didn't care.

So when I returned to the Canadian Cannabis Clinic for my follow-up appointment, I explained that because of my disabilities, I did not want to get into making my own witch's brew; it would be much safer to obtain pre-made cannabis oil, and therefore, change my medical supplier to CanniMed.

"Oh, of course! You could have called us to come back sooner! We always suggest the butter recipe first because cost is often pro-hibitive for so many patients."

It is indeed quite costly, and there's no health insurance coverage for medical marijuana, except to claim it as an annual medical expense on your income tax. Years later, I now get a "compassionate pricing" discount with Tilray, another cannabis supplier, because I receive a Canada Pension Disability Benefit.

I also had to sign a document agreeing that I would not operate a motor vehicle until at least six hours after dosing.

So, nervously, at 7 a.m. on Valentine's Day, 2016, I dropped .3 millilitres of the foul-tasting liquid under my tongue from the plastic syringe provided for my first legal dose of cannabis oil. "Start low and go slow" were the instructions repeated everywhere. I also read that it could take anywhere from half an hour to two hours before any effects might be felt, if it all. If I didn't feel any different, I was to wait at least four hours before taking any more.

For me, the results were miraculous.

Within 15 minutes, my right arm and leg felt slightly less seized. And when I took my bedtime dose, I was asleep within half an hour, whereas some nights I would thrash about all night because there was always something hurting somewhere.

My pharmacist at the time, from Rexall, wrote a wonderful letter to my family doctor proposing a schedule for me to wean off the morphine while increasing my cannabis oil intake. And it worked! With the collaboration of the Canadian Cannabis Clinic, Dr. Linney and the pharmacist, I slowly reduced the morphine until I finally no longer needed the opiate.

And not just morphine. Baclophen, my antispasticity drug, got the boot too; I reduced my intake of migraine-reducing pregabalin by almost half, and with a mug of warm lemon water every morning, I no longer needed the godawful Metamucil or colon self-massaging (thanks, Jen Spak, RMT & Osteopath); and I even reduced my intake of magnesium glycinate (thanks, Sara Vadeboncoeur, ND) because my digestion worked so much better.

My lower bodily functions improved even more from pelvic

physiotherapy, (thanks, Andrea Plitz, PT, RYT and co-founder, Bloom Integrative Health and Movement Centre), along with regular neurophysiotherapy tune-ups, (thanks, Lucie Hemstead), which helped calm many of my worst patterning issues from the strokes, allowing me to move more freely. More movement; less chronic pain.

With my spasticity reduced by the cannabis oil, I was walking like a gazelle now – faster, farther and with less pain, and the group of my "fabulous five" female health practitioners, who intimately understood my complex issues, continue to be my life coaches, helping me maintain my strengthened synergies to this day. (Dr. Linney has since retired from her general practice, replaced by the ever-amiable Dr. Elie Skaff. He is an equally fabulous-five contributor.)

I try to walk at least 30 minutes a day, even if it's broken up into three 10-minute sessions. I wear a water CamelBak (a hydration backpack) with a nozzle to suck from, so that I don't have to interrupt my momentum on my weaker right side while my left hand struggles to open a water bottle. The weight on my back also helps anchor me and better balance my stride.

The crappier I feel, the more important it is to walk. Moving frees me. The first 10 minutes are always the hardest, but then, when my joints are lubricated, and I've burned off all the protesting lactic acid, (as Dr. Skaff explained), a new rhythm sets in. I have lots of tricks to keep me motivated. Even on my favourite routes, I try not to go the same way twice. I love walking in different neighbourhoods, on streets where I've never been before, because then my focus is on what I'm discovering, not on how I'm feeling. I can go beyond looking down to check where my feet are. And as a nature lover, I won't hesitate to pause to snap a few pics with my mobile phone. That way, I don't need a "rest" break. I'm literally just stopping to smell the roses. In winter, when it's cold and potentially icy, I will drive to a safer place. I tried mall walking, but I hate it. Not enough sunshine and oxygen and nothing to see except window after window of stupid stuff that nearly nobody needs. After 10 or 15 minutes driving with the seat heater on, my buns become nice and toasty, and I can't wait to work off the heat.

* * *

I am a firm believer that after a stroke, recovery is not limited to two years. Recovery never stops, as long as you keep working at it. If I can keep my mind open to receiving new stimuli, and if I keep feeding it different things to process, it's amazing how much it can adapt and figure out how to do things differently.

For example, when I first started my yoga routine, I could not keep my balance without wearing aqua shoes for extra support. However, after years and years of rolling around on the carpeted floor in our master bedroom, focussing on moving with lightness and intuitive movements (and fantasizing that I was a ballerina), I found that certain positions, such as the child pose or kneeling, transitioned to actually becoming easier and less painful barefoot, without the encumbrance of shoes. Then I discovered other positions could work a little better by adding just a pair of socks, such as bridging (lying on the floor with knees bent and lifting my back off the floor up to the neck). It may not be the brain that's improving, but little by little, by changing my physical habits, I try to give my brain (and therefore my affected body parts) new processing signals. Every little bit helps. For me, by doing something a little differently every day, even something as simple as changing one aspect of my daily routine, like the order of my morning self-care tasks – helps with neuroplasticity.

If I try something and fail, I try again. And again. If it still does not work, can I figure out a different way to do it? And if I still can't do it, how important is it to me? Can I forget about it, or should I find someone to help out? I always try to assess the risks before I attempt anything new, even though I set myself up for failure or injury sometimes. But even when I fail, I always try to celebrate the small victories.

26

Kayaking, Snowshoeing
and Using Good Props

A huge testament to the success of my intuitive rolling around and stretching on the floor year after year is that I've taught myself how to roll out of a kayak on a floating dock, like a harp seal.

When I first broached the idea of kayaking with my daughter and husband, they adamantly wailed NO, NO, NO!

My daughter worried what could happen if my kayak flipped and I couldn't get out. She was probably picturing a traditional small-holed kayak that would indeed pose much more of a risk. Now, however, the variety of large, open-mouthed, inflatable, foldable kayaks and sailboards is infinitesimal.

"I'd wear a lifejacket, and I can swim well enough to free myself," I insisted.

I'd been doing light aquafit classes in warm water twice a week since 1992, and I could now swim across the exercise pool, front-crawl style, holding my breath with my head underwater. Nothing feels better than having a good swim, followed by a hot shower; every cell of my body gets activated and then radiates energy.

Jean-Pierre insisted he accompany me the first time. We went to Oziles' Marina at Petrie Island, a beautiful crisscrossing of sand dunes and wooded peninsulas on the Ottawa River, and only a 10-minute drive from our home in Orléans. Recently christened a municipal ecological reserve, with its gorgeous sandy beaches, picturesque trails and abundant wildlife, it's a community treasure.

After we paid for one hour and collected our life jackets, oars and safety kits, a shy young marina hand accompanied us down to the wharf to help us get into our kayaks. I went first, getting on my hands and knees, then swinging around to sit down sideways on the edge of the deck. (Thanks again, yoga!) With the two strong men holding the kayak close while doing everything they could to support me, I extended my stronger left leg outward and clumsily plopped down several feet into the seat of the large opening, then found my lethargic right leg, and hauled it into place.

"Okay!" I shouted happily. "I'm in!" What a feeling of exhilaration.

JP got into his kayak with a lot less fanfare, and our next big challenge was to figure out how to paddle our way through the thin channel to avoid colliding with a variety of leisure and fishing crafts to reach more open water. After a few random circles with the paddles, we figured out how they worked, and so we bumbled along, butting against some of the boat piers with glee as we cleared the channel.

I started pointing all over the place with my oar. "Wow! Look at all the beautiful birds!"

Swallows swung through the air at random, gobbling insects. Mama ducks nestled with their fuzzy little ducklings, hugging yellowy reeds and bright green lily pads near the shoreline. Later, a great blue heron swept right past us, landing amongst the reeds. Glorious!

The inlet we paddled through had no current, but as we neared the mouth of the Ottawa River, the increasing swells from a passing motorboat tossed our kayaks around like baby toys in a bathtub – freaking us out a bit, being the fresh paddlers that we were. We had no intention of capsizing the first time on the water, so we turned ourselves around and retreated as quickly as we could to another quieter inlet amongst the beautiful wetlands. Heavenly.

The hardest part came next. How the heck was I going to get out of my kayak?

The drop down from the deck to the kayak was over a foot. I tried, but there was no way I could independently hoist myself out. Fortunately, the shy young assistant mariner was around to give JP enough moral support to successfully get up and exit on his own. Then finally, after much dilly-dallying on my part to find the best orientation for the kayak – followed by too much pulling and forcing on their part – the two of them managed to lug me upwards and drag me out, feet flailing.

"Oh … wow," I gasped. "That was fantastic! … No, no, it's okay." I batted their hands away. "Let me get up on my own … "

Even back then, yoga poses helped me right myself, using the table and downward-dog asanas (body postures) to get back up to a standing position. We were both exhausted, but I was nonetheless grinning from ear to ear. However, I was already thinking about how to improve things next time. I didn't want JP to blow his aorta being so physical and anxious over my wellbeing, though.

"Next time, I'll beach the kayak on that gravel hill back there for the bigger boat launch, and then I can just roll out on my side. I think that would be much easier."

And yes, it was for me, but not for poor Jean-Pierre. The hill was so steep I couldn't get my kayak high enough out of the water to roll out on my own, so JP had to get out of his kayak to pull mine up, spot me while I thrashed around figuring out which way to do my turtle crawl exit and then stand myself up. Then JP had to get back into his kayak and paddle some more to the dock and get out, while I trooped back to the marina shed through the lot reserved for the larger craft. Hmm, that was also a wee bit too exhausting.

The young Oziles' mariner was upset with us for leaving the kayak at the launch for the larger boats, which was not part of the rental facility. So next time, after JP helped me beach the kayak and exit, I attached my kayak to his so that he could tow it back to the rental dock. It still seemed to be way too much exertion for him though, especially for a guy with two leaking heart valves, after contracting rheumatic fever and almost dying as a teenager.

Next time, we tried the same process a few more times from an even wackier steep, rocky hill with a bit more flat land at the bottom that was closer to the launch, but I found the climb up the hill uncomfortably perilous.

I finally decided (at least then) that our Petrie Island experience was officially over, after poor Poppa Hen capsized when jockeying the two kayaks back to the dock amongst a large group of people. This was particularly embarrassing for him. However, I did manage to resuscitate his waterlogged cell phone by covering it in a bowl of rice for three days.

We enjoyed relocating to beautiful Dow's Lake, paddling past the Dominion Arboretum at the Central Experimental Farm, and all the way to the historic Rideau Canal, a UNESCO World Heritage site, and to the Rideau River locks near Carleton University. Carleton's big strong, "he-man" summer students who worked at the marina expertly plucked me out and onto their floating deck, which was almost at water level, making the process a piece of cake.

I still kept dreaming about kayaking back at Petrie Island, though. It was such a rare, beautiful spot, and so close to our home. The newly created municipal park and ecological conservation area offered a free public boat launch, complete with a ramp and a beach, located near picnic tables bordering spectacular trails amid lagoons. Maybe we could get inflatable kayaks; they wouldn't have to be mounted on top of our little car – or maybe one day, the existing private company on site, Oziles' Marina, where rented kayaks were available, would fix up its boat launch and relocate it to the other side of the inlet, which opened up directly to a myriad of lagoons and a wide, calm inner waterway.

And whaddayaknow, three years later, the marina was sold, becoming the Petrie Island Marina, and the new owners rebuilt a whole new facility – yes, on the other side of the inlet, closer to the lagoons, and in their fourth year of operation, I noticed they had added a floating dock!

In the meantime, every morning, I continued to do my own intuitive morning yoga, always rolling back and forth and then boomeranging from top to bottom on the floor, making as much contact as possible on my affected side to stimulate it and remind my brain that every prickly sensation comes from places that can still move and help me out.

I knew I could kayak at Petrie Island now. I didn't care if I got wet. JP, as always, worried that I was overestimating myself, but I persuaded him that I had to try. And I was right. Easy peasy! I got in with only JP holding the kayak for me. The vistas were breath-taking, as we paddled around lily pads, purple, pink and white water flowers, herons and egrets, bullfrogs with their green, brown-spotted rotund bellies, turtles stretching out their necks while soaking in the sun on exposed logs, and a slick, lightning-fast otter shooting past … everything I'd dreamed of.

And it turned out that I rolled out of the kayak faster than JP did. (He claims the apple in his pocket slowed him down. Yeah, yeah.) Anyway, while he held onto my craft, I leaned over to my right, grounding myself, took a deep breath, then swung my stronger left leg over and pushed down hard, rolling out and flipping all the way over until I was safely on deck on my stomach.

"Wow! That was so good! Need help to stand up?"

"Nope – I got this."

Then I tabled onto my hands and knees, toed up into a triangular downward-dog position and then, keeping my core strong, knees slightly bent, slowly raised myself on the perpetually moving, floating deck to an unsteady standing position, grinning from ear to ear. JP gawked at me in disbelief.

What a rush!

* * *

Recently, I went kayaking solo at Petrie Island. The new owners, probably observing the increasing number of customers with burgeoning bellies and increasingly poor docking skills, had now constructed a large, sturdy wooden deck at water level that their kayaks sit on. Now, all we have to do is get into the kayak right on the deck, and one of the friendly staff just pushes you out, and upon your return, they just pull you back in.

Sometimes dreams do come true …

* * *

JP and I also love to snowshoe, especially amidst Petrie's forested trails.

We got our first low-cost snowshoes, and they were fine, in the beginning. I needed JP to help me secure them from time to time, but once his hands got too cold after fiddling with his buckles and then mine, it ruined his own pleasurable experience. (JP is always freezing, while I'm a perennial post-menopausal hot mess.) I warned him that I was going to invest in a better pair for myself, and he should too.

In the meantime, I took a few serious tumbles. I had to learn the hard way to always hold my snowshoe poles far away from my feet and be at least mildly conscious of where all my body parts were with every movement, before going too far or too long, when fatigue or distraction could cause a wipeout from a loss of balance. I've learned a few tricks, like giving my right arm a rest by letting the pole trail behind me and using only my left arm for a few paces where the land is level and well packed with snow. Often, I'll need to stop and readjust my right hand's grip through the pole strap, as it often comes loose during the exertion. My gloves are always flexible leather because I find they provide better traction.

When I became confident that I wanted to continue snowshoeing, I upgraded to the perfect pair. They require only one hand to secure the foot. All I have to do is insert my foot into its acrylic sheath, pre-laced with a coated wire, then turn the good-sized knob to tighten the sheath to my liking and – bingo! I got game! And on my own.

Independence: That's Living …

The following winter, JP decided to scale up too, and he was delighted. Since he could put on his snowshoes so much quicker and didn't have to worry about helping me, he had more energy to enjoy our adventures, and best of all, his hands didn't get as cold. For several years now, we have enjoyed snowshoeing so much more because the new gear has made it easier, more comfortable and safer, too. I think I've wiped out only once since my snowshoe upgrade.

It is so important to find the right athletic equipment that suits your individual needs if you want to enjoy your pastime.

Yoga props (such as blocks or wedges) are another example. At first, I hated using any kind of prop because breaking away to go get it and then trying to place it where it was supposed to go would often exhaust me and completely disrupt my meditative efforts.

For example, after successfully using the Theraball for a great deal of pain relief, I bought a hard-foam yoga brick to sit on in the lotus position to allow my arms to hang freely without touching the floor. I wanted to improve my posture and deep breathing.

It took me a couple of years just to figure out how to seat myself on top of the brick. Sometimes, I would twist the wrong way and hurt myself, so for a while, I temporarily abandoned it as a silly, "thick-as-a-brick" idea, just like trying to kayak at Petrie Island.

However, everything suddenly clicked. My girlfriend from Grade 6, Karen Titus, who also enjoys yoga, showed me a soft, but firm, long and wide, rectangular back bolster (a firm support prop) that her partner Doug Smale brought home one day. I immediately ordered one on Amazon.

It was blissful just to lie on it, shoulders and arms falling gently over its sides, palms facing upwards, resting on the soft carpet, and opening the chest and letting it rise and fall, just breathing.

In Bob Dylan's song, *Idiot Wind,* he sings, "It's a wonder that you still know how to breathe." Actually, most of us don't know how to breathe properly. And even if we've learned a little, and practised a lot, it can remain a tough challenge. Especially when you're in chronic pain.

After years and years of coaching in pelvic physiotherapy, yoga and meditation, I still find it difficult to just breathe, and think about nothing else. Most of us almost never use our lungs to our full capacity. We breathe quickly and shallowly, or we hold our breath and don't even realize we've stopped breathing.

I do that all the time. Another dear friend from Grade 6, Glenda

Quaile, who's a retired professor of nursing living in the Vancouver area, has barked "CATHY – BREATHE!" at me on more than one occasion when I'm excited and yapping on and on about something – it's so easy to forget to breathe!

Breathing is the best way to pause, open up the channels in your body, relax and relieve the tightness that contributes to discomfort. It's one of the few things you can do on your own at any time to regain control of whatever's plaguing you. Even if you hurt all over, you're unable to move, you're dead tired, or nearly catatonic with grief or despair, you still must breathe. When you breathe from your solar plexus to whatever part of you that needs it most, you feed your heart and your brain, and from there, you can go wherever you want to go, at least in your mind, so you start to experience the joys of meditation. Soft or thrumming background music can also be calming or invigorating, depending on your mood. JP makes me playlists of songs I danced to in high school. Meditation apps can be extremely helpful to guide breathing and address your daily goals. Right now I am delighted with an app that provides gorgeous, uplifting 12-minute musical interludes, combined with 10 Hz square waveform frequencies, many which are inaudible to the human ear, that have apparently been proven by NASA research to increase the growth of stem cells, enhance cellular proliferation genes, and downgrade 175 aging genes, whatever that means … Maybe it doesn't really work, but it sure makes me feel ecstatic …

And if nothing works that day, try a vibrator.

27

On Falling

Today, as we age, we are bombarded with cautionary advice about how to minimize various risks to avoid falls. "Don't have rugs you might trip on, use correct support when you need it, wear supportive shoes, yada yada yada … "

With my skewed proprioception, it's always a conscious struggle to visually check out exactly where half my body parts are before doing anything. So over the last 40-some years, I have inadvertently become an expert on falling.

I lose and correct my balance several times a day, giving JP constant fits of protective anxiety whenever he notices my arms flying up to steady myself. This fragile equilibrium gives me advance warning to realize when I've exceeded my tipping point though, and I've learned it's better not to fight it.

Ooops, you're going down … gently bring your arms inward,

let yourself collapse softly, and keep your head up befo-
WHOOMPH!

Ooof! Still in one piece? … Okay! Well, that was an adventure …

* * *

In the shower, I usually keep my eyes closed. Vision can be a distraction when I have to concentrate my focus on understanding all the altered sensations coursing through me so I can keep my feet stable on a slippery surface. Our grab bar is vertical because moving my arm straight up and down requires less guessing for me than the traditional angled alignment. I also find it more stabilizing to feel for the tap, shower head and shampoo with my fully functional left hand, as opposed to opening my eyes and instinctively turning myself toward whatever I'm after, which risks my numb foot moving imperceptibly. I also have a shower chair to take breaks, do bathtub yoga, or shower completely seated on days when I'm not at my best.

* * *

Buying anything for my feet is always a hassle. I can't tell how my right foot feels in the shoe until it's been on my foot for a long time. If I'm at a shoe store, I don't even try them on anymore. I take them home to do extensive experimentation. In order to keep new footwear, orthotics, or even new socks, I need to have them pass several test walks indoors, on different surfaces, at different times of day, before they are deemed worthy to try outdoors. Some days, the foot stings more than usual, and because it can't feel anything but heat, cold and pain, it takes much longer to figure out what's going on. I'll watch myself walk in a mirror. If I'm having any doubts, a foot inspection may reveal red or swollen areas that indicate too much friction or pressure. And if it's too much of a struggle to force and yank the immobile foot into the exact position before exhaustion results, it's a no-go. The footwear gets returned.

I learned these valuable lessons very quickly one hot, sunny morning with the first step I took outside the back entrance of the Rehabilitation Centre. I was returning to my car after getting some new customized orthotics inserted into a brand new, bouncy pair of running shoes with "reflexive" soles. One step out the door sent me flying, my bare knees and wrists crashing down onto the searing hot pavement. Lots of painful, bloody scratches. Nothing broken though. I limped back to the car, which of course was parked far, far away in order to maximize an expected pleasant walk in the spirit of a rehabilitative adventure.

That was how I learned not to fight a fall.

* * *

Over the years, I've broken all five toes on my right foot, though not at the same time. I didn't even realize I had previously broken my four smaller toes until after another fall, when X-rays confirmed that I had fractured the big toe.

I most likely broke the first four in a dark hotel corridor in Toronto, early one morning. JP and I were in an excited rush to check out, on our way to the glorious sand-dune beaches of Sandbanks Provincial Park. I should have known better not to try to carry a take-out coffee in my trustworthy hand and pull a small suitcase in the other. Anyway, two steps out the door and I wiped out, the coffee splashing everywhere except on me, with a nasty abrasion on the outside of my knee that wouldn't stop bleeding. Somehow, the front desk got me some ice and several bandages, and I made it to the underground parking lot, nursing my wounds.

"That's it! We're going back home to Ottawa," JP said sourly.

"No! I'll be fine!"

I won the argument, and so off we went to Prince Edward County. With a cane that I always keep in the car, just in case, we navigated between the flattest sand dunes to the beach, and I had a wonderful time lying down and doing absolutely nothing.

And now when we go to the beach, I use a pool noodle as a cane to make my way through the hot sand, since I'm going to be floating on it in the water. One less thing to carry. Simple is best.

* * *

However, my most recent adventure in August 2022 was not quite like the others.

I was on my way to visit my dear brother Fred Roberts, who was in palliative care at, of all coincidences, good old Saint-Vincent Hospital. He was born with the same heart defect as my mom, and suffered numerous cardiac arrests, thankfully rescued by the pacemaker-defibrillator after miraculously surviving his first heart stoppage at age 47. (Some off-duty firefighters with their life-saving cardiac resuscitation paddles just happened to be in the same Farm Boy parking lot where he was waiting to pick up his daughter after finishing her shift.) But that wasn't his only curse. It wouldn't be long now before his lungs were rendered incapable of drawing breath from terminal idiopathic pulmonary fibrosis … and he would be granted medical assistance in dying –

WHAM!

Suddenly my face slammed into the sidewalk, bruising my nose, swelling my upper lip, and leaving front teeth jangling. Luckily, the meatiest part of my face absorbed the impact. I didn't feel concussed and nothing felt broken.

Still face-first on the ground, half on the grass and half on the sidewalk, I could see my glasses off to the right, and felt my left hearing aid fly off with the glasses.

Shit, where did the stupid little grey thing go? My blurry eyes searched while I figured out the best way to get on my hands and knees.

Ooooh! My left knee screamed.

Aghh, shit … my good hand …

The fourth and fifth digits of my now dominant left hand were scraped raw in spots and bleeding, with the pinkie skewed at an impossible angle, and I watched an ominous nodule bloat upwards between the two end fingers into the shape of a cone with the diameter of a Toonie, right before my eyes.

Never mind. Must get up. Now. I positioned my uninjured fingers and palms on the ground *(ow ow ow)* and brought my left knee forward to initiate the struggle to get on my feet, and let my head and arms hang down like a ragdoll for a few moments to get my bearings before rising completely upright. Odd drops of blood still plopped onto the sidewalk.

Jesus, what have you done to yourself this time?

Slowly, I raised my head and looked around. *Get your glasses first so you can find the stupid hearing aid …* With trepidation, I carefully sidestepped to the right, leaned down as far as I could, and watched my trembling right finger clumsily latch on to an arm of the teal-coloured glasses that nearly matched the colour of the grass.

Aha! Now, get them back on your head without bleeding all over yourself. Clearer vision returned. *Okay, good. Now where'd that little hearing aid bugger go?*

I scanned the ground in front of me. The sidewalk was empty. *It must be buried in the grass somewhere … can't see it, though …*

A feeling of panic began to rise in my throat.

I surveyed my surroundings. I was alone …

Aha! There's my wee friend!

* * *

My family doctor suggested I think about getting a walker, but my physiotherapist and I knew that a walker would change my gait, so we all agreed it was time to begrudgingly use my friend, the cane, whenever I leave the house.

This fall gave me a horrible scare. It crushed my confidence and making the conscious decision to go back to using my cane all the time deeply depressed me.

I'm starting to fail … Lately, I'd become a bit more light-headed than usual when I stood up too quickly and more unsteady on my feet.

I was ordered to stop taking cannabis oil for a week to reboot my system so that I would require a smaller dose when I resumed, and my cannabis prescription would not be renewed until my family doctor checked out my blood pressure and made sure I didn't have arrhythmia. Dr. Skaff had me start using a blood pressure monitor at home to see whether any of my medications needed adjustment. Ah, the joys of aging …

You gotta go slower than slow, right now. And you need your cane to always remind you of that. It has regained its status as your essential four-season friend.

So now, keeping my cane by my side awards me more freedom. A conversation with my dear friend Lucie Delorme reminded me that as we age, there are more and more changes happening at a time when it becomes harder and harder to accept them. Aging gracefully is far, far better and safer than refusing to embrace your limitations; by accepting them, you can still do things you never thought possible.

No one wants to break a hip, or die from a head injury.

28

Climbing The Acropolis

I have always loved to travel. As a child, I enjoyed spectacular family camping road trips across Canada and the U.S., to Banff, Yellowstone, Glacier National Park, and Tofino, on the west coast of Vancouver Island, at a time when the only access was a perilous gravel road, and we were towing a wooden fold-down trailer that my father had built himself. Those were the best family times I remember when my brother Fred and I were kids.

I got hooked on international travel at 15, when I flew for the first time to Paris along with Dave Tod, from the same high school as me, and other Ottawa teens (selected by their French teachers as being most likely to become bilingual) on a mind-blowing, three-week student exchange. We were billetted with families living in Les Clayes-sous-Bois, an ancient village originating from the 12th century, not far from Paris. And the following summer, many of its teenagers came to stay with our families. Many romances stood the test of time, (including mine, with the heart-stopping Alain Jarrossay, R.I.P.), and lifelong friendships continue to this day.

During the summer I graduated from Grade 12, my long-time girlfriend Julie Cobb and I loved to travel so much that we even signed up for interviews at the Chateau Laurier to become flight attendants for Air Canada. (I'm sure we were screened out because we were too young, though – ha ha.)

* * *

The strokes have never stopped me from travelling, either. Just being in a new place, experiencing all the different sites – the people, how they dress, their cultures and the varied architecture, feeling the different weather, hearing everything from subdued beats to the yawning roars of ocean waves, smelling its sweet salty scent – enjoying the aromas of different vegetation – heck, even exhaust fumes shimmering in the heat during horrendous traffic jams, savouring delicious foreign cuisines – and it's never enough – all of life everywhere fills my heart.

We have all heard or experienced horror stories about airline delays, cancellations, lost luggage or getting bumped, especially with the added restraints due to the COVID-19 pandemic, but as a person with disabilities, I can honestly say that all but one airline I've used has done everything they can to treat me with respect and consideration.

However, you must take extra time to do the homework before you book your flight. Every airline has its own system of accommodating requests for assistance. They need to know right away if you plan to bring your own wheelchair or some sort of assistive device that is essential for your well-being (say a breathing device or a support dog, for example) and there may be limitations. Can it fit in overhead storage, or is it too large or fragile to be checked as baggage? If so, there may be required forms to complete and have signed beforehand. Also, does the particular plane you plan to book have adequate space to accommodate this device? Special seating or seat selection will likely cost extra, if it can be provided. If you have any doubts, ask away until you are satisfied. Compare it to what other airlines offer, if you have a choice.

For boarding assistance at the airport, also mention this to whomever is booking your flight. Do you need a wheelchair escort from check-in right to the waiting area outside the gate? Do you also require wheelchair assistance from the gate to board the plane? As a rule I say yes to everything because gates can always get changed at the last minute. Even a standard gate may have an extremely long gangway that may curve or change elevation significantly, so be sure you ask the agent who brings you from security to the gate about the geography from the gate to the plane. On a busy day, unless you speak up, the wheelchair may not be left at the gate for the early boarding call if the agent needs to hurry off to use it somewhere else. Boarding assistance can get complicated for the airlines, so it's important to follow up with them yourself a few days before your flight leaves to ensure that it's properly noted what sort of assistance you'll need.

There are two fantastic things about wheelchair assistance that make all the difference in withstanding air travel. First, you and your companion get to skip the line for the security screenings, and two: neither of you have to worry about finding your way through an airport you're unfamiliar with, since the agents know exactly where they are taking you.

This was particularly true when JP and I had to change planes in Frankfurt International Airport on our way to Barcelona, Spain. In order to bypass the stairs and escalators to reach our appropriate gate, we were blessed to have an agent dipsy-doodle us through a labyrinth of lengthy corridors, up-and-down elevators and connecting annexes. We never could have managed to negotiate such a complicated route by ourselves.

And do use the same line of thinking when booking places to stay. If it's a multilevel building, is there an elevator? If not, can you reserve one on the ground floor? Do you need a room that accommodates a wheelchair, including the shower?

* * *

In October 2018, JP and I travelled to Greece, and we spent three days in Athens before ferrying to the islands of Mykonos and Santorini. My ultimate goal was to scale the Acropolis, stand on top of the world, and marvel at our privilege to be on this beautiful planet.

On our last morning in Athens, when we were scheduled to make the ascent, I woke up with a crushing migraine headache. I couldn't hide it from Jean-Pierre, and while I was sitting on the toilet, head down, massaging my eyelids and temples, I could hear JP anxiously muttering, "Oh no … I knew this was going to happen, I knew it, I knew it."

All of a sudden I heard myself ordering him to "STOP IT. WE.

ARE. GOING, OK?"

"Yeah, but what about our reservation tonight for the Michelin Restaurant I made over a month ago?"

"Please don't argue. You're just making it worse. We are doing the Acropolis. No discussion. It's still early. We'll leave now. We'll link arms till we get to the top."

I managed to keep down a coffee and some kind of dry puff-pastry, and we were off, as it's best to get there as early in the morning as possible. Fewer crowds. Less heat.

We hopped onto the red double-decker tourist bus right in front of our hotel, and hopped off a few blocks later. A very short ride.

In silence, we handed in our tickets, waited in the cue, and when our time came, we began our ascent.

There is an elevator, but it must be reserved a day in advance, and even then, there is still no guarantee it will be available. Besides, we wanted the real experience.

There can be shutdowns to the site if the weather gets too hot. Fortunately, it was a warm, clear, sunny morning.

Even when dry, the some-200 irregular, steep stone stairs leading to the summit have been buffed to a shiny glaze, like polished marble, from the footsteps of millions of peoples who've made this trek for almost 2,500 years, both to build and worship from this iconic citadel that looks down from the skies.

If it rains, those who have previously booked tickets must be extremely careful. Many have experienced serious falls and injuries.

There were firm metal bars on each side of the stairs. When no one was on their way down, JP would tuck my cane under his arm and I would grab the left stairwell, my right arm woven loosely inside JP's arm, while he held onto the railing on his side. When we saw someone coming, I'd take my cane back from JP, squeeze next to him, and wait for them to pass. Whenever there was constant descending traffic, we would continue upwards together, arms tightly wound with us sandwiched together, me breathing deep in time with every step, with my cane in my left hand to steady me. Sometimes, the stairs would turn abruptly at right angles, so we would wait till it was all clear, then Jean-Pierre would edge me over to whatever uneven side's railing that would work best for me to hang onto to while using my cane with the other hand, and prop me up as equally as possible on the other side. During these maneuvers, it was obvious to "the others" that they needed to pause until I'd safely navigated the turn.

There were a few spots along the way to stop for a while and revel in the gorgeous views of other ancient structures, desert-like vegetation amongst the huge stones that resembled lunar rocks, and the endless azure Mediterranean skies. It was so easy to appreciate how this awe-inspiring beauty led the early Greeks to create mythologies based on all-powerful Gods to try to make sense of it all.

Finally, we took our last step to the top.

Eureka!

I felt so blessed just to be there, let alone awed by the magnificence, especially after all the difficulties we had surmounted.

With a huge smile, I placed my arms around my husband (nearly caning him), and we held each other close. "Thank you," I murmured into his shoulder.

The Acropolis itself was roped off and scaffolded on one side, as restoration efforts continue almost constantly. The level of degradation alarmed me. It was warm, but the wind gusts were chilly. We spent almost an hour strolling around roped-off debris and other structures scattered on top of the same crest as the Acropolis. In spite of the growing crowds, it truly felt like we were amidst an archeological miracle.

The steep descent was equally challenging. I was never quite sure how my right foot would land on each step until it was placed there, so I had to be vigilant, one step at a time. My legs were getting shaky.

Oh, so glad … we're almost back to the bottom… I really don't feel well … not too much farther …

Fortunately, there was always a bright-red tour bus waiting or on the way, and it wasn't long before we boarded, save for an extremely rude woman who butted in front of us right at the door to get the best seat in the otherwise empty bus. I almost lost my balance, as she swiped past us without even a nod or a smile.

We sat ourselves towards the back of the bus, and as soon as it lurched down the hill, I threw up a long, messy stream into the aisle. JP secretly giggled to himself as the vomit trickled towards the front, right to the shoes at the spot where the unsuspecting rude woman sat …

Come on … I didn't do it on purpose …

* * *

Sadly, we didn't make it to the Michelin-starred restaurant that night. JP was very glum about that, and he wandered about the agora near our hotel while I lay listlessly in our dark hotel room, and we moved out onto the tiny balcony together once the sun had gone down. He ate a crummy gyro, while I sipped on ginger ale and a few biscuits, waiting for my head to clear. I had no trouble soothing myself, though. Even though I was out of action, I was so happy. After all, there are many, many Michelin restaurants around the world, but only one Acropolis …

And together, we did it!

I had come so far from those early days after my first stroke, and then my second. Through perseverance and resilience, and the love of my family, I had made it to the top of this iconic monument. It was a peak moment.

What a triumph.

Next time, the Egyptian Pyramids, maybe … probably have missed my chance to take on Machu Picchu …

29

Coming Full Circle

While we've lived with the COVID-19 pandemic for four years, it feels like I've aged a decade.

On Father's Day 2021, with a lull between the second and third pandemic wave (or was it the third or fourth?), which required either quarantining or self-isolation, my daughter and her hubby buoyed us with an invitation to their gorgeous cottage to honour our patriarch, Jean-Pierre.

We successfully navigated the drive, climbing around craggy rock hills before hanging a sharp left turn just past the crest of a steep downslope. This led to a soft and narrow, rocky earthen lane, down, down, down through forest … and as we rounded another perilous turn, the trees peeked open just enough to reveal a breathtaking panorama of a heavily forested island, its dark, jagged rock rising up from a massive, deep blue lake.

As always, once we were over the combined thrill and trepidation of the descent, a long, wide, deck-like stairway with two landings welcomed us. The entrance, adorned by seasonal blooms planted in a small, wooden wheelbarrow next to the stairdeck's cliffside fence, beckoned us further down through the forest.

Even descending the staircase was a spectacular treat – we saw their beach area with its outdoor fireplace, the glorious sundeck jutting out over the water, with the hot tub, dock and motorboat peeking through the cedar, pine and birch branches, the scented breezes whispering "this is heaven" …

By the time we reached the front porch, my daughter was already waiting for her retired parents, greeting us with a small, content smile. She took some of our things and urged us inside. And her husband, all smiles, came over from the kitchen to greet us as well. Lots of hugs and kisses.

The view from the entirely windowed southwest corner of their second home revealed a private cove, the island, some arms of the lake and expanses of hilly pristine forest farther away. It was easy to become so transfixed by the spectacular panorama that I could forget to be mindful of my footing so as not to tumble down the fairly hefty, eight-inch step into the lower-level large sitting room and dining area.

We all got cozy on the L-shaped couch with warm mugs of coffee and chatted until her cat, named "Brother," slowly waltzed into view. (Since our daughter was an only child, his name made complete sense.)

Brother is a huge, stupidly erratic and lovable tabby, but he can also be brooding and occasionally vicious, when not in the mood to socialize. On that day, he was very well-behaved though, and happy to play the role assigned to him.

Among the cats our daughter had previously force-dressed in Cabbage Patch Kids outfits, old crocheted baby sets or Halloween costumes as a little girl, Brother was the most compliant. He wore his costumes proudly. He loved to sleep in piles of torn tissue paper and bows after any gifting festivities, and for the last several years, he lorded over us wearing his kingly Christmas mane – a red and green, layered fishnet neck wreath, adorned with tiny sparkly silver bells. He also loved to lap up the pine water from Christmas trees.

That day, Brother sported a long, white cotton undershirt yanked down over two thirds of his girth. Our son-in-law quickly straightened it as their frequently fat-shamed cat lumbered past, and for the first time, I could see some writing on the tank top. It was upside down, and skewed …

Wait … Soon … to be … a … Big Brother … ???

My eyes flipped over to meet my daughter's. Hers were beaming with joy.

"What – are you pregnant?"

"YES!" Our arms flew around each other. "Oh my God, honey!" I gushed into her shoulder. "Oh, I'm so, so happy for you!"

The men joined in our joyful embrace.

In January 2023, my darling daughter gave birth to her own perfect little girl. Becoming a grandmother has given me even more magical reasons to stick around as long as possible.

30

No

As of March 2023, over 6.5 million Canadians do not have access to primary health care, and the COVID-19 pandemic has blown the lid off the already crippled infrastructure of our healthcare system. It's utterly frightening. Every day, JP and I dread more and more that our caring family doctor will decide he's fed up, throw in the towel on his general practice, and switch to a less stressful and more rewarding field of medicine.

These days, by the time I wake up and find my way to the bathroom, I'm already feeling overwhelmed. It takes me so long to poop, get myself dosed, dressed and stretched that I'm already exhausted by the time I'm ready to descend on the stairlift to the main floor. All I can think is *how am I going to make it through the day?*

I find it always helps to have my next day planned out the night before. It provides motivation and clues about how I should dress. The next morning, I'll check the weather and my iPhone calendar as soon as I'm safely perched on the throne.

Alright … yes, you're doing this today …

On a morning when I don't know what I'm doing, anxiety rages through my chest. I have no idea what clothes to put on. What hurts the most today? And how bad am I burning and sweating, and where? I'll often spend an hour (or two) on the ensuite throne, checking our volatile weather, my calendar, the news headlines, my email, Facebook and lastly, feeding my addiction to playing solitaire and other games, while I wait until the meds have kicked in and I'm comfortably numb enough to think straight. On a really bad day, I go straight to gaming. Often I don't even try to poop until after I've figured out what the day's plan will be; then my body parts will start to unseize and tell me *okay, now you know the plan, so time to get going …*

Even going for a neighbourhood stroll can upset me now. Struggling to get out the front door before the heat or the cold or the more violent winds become unbearable; seeing all the pines and firs dying, plus all the weakened ones flattened or bent by the recent derecho – a line of brutally intense, rapidly moving and damaging windstorms and thunderstorms across a wide area – a direct consequence of climate change and a visual slap in the face that our world is dying, and there's so little I can do about it.

Even when I'm doing my morning meditative yogic stretch routine, my view through the window shows me a tall, bashed up and bent pine tree, permanently leaning eastward, its needles thrashed bare in places.

Aging can suck in so many ways.

31

Yes

While some mornings I wake up feeling so overwhelmed it's a struggle to function, most days, I can seize enough optimism to repeat to myself it's going to be a great day.

I wake up at 4:30 a.m. to tinkle. *Ahhh …* JP keeps saying he wants me to join him in bed early those mornings before he gets up for his first tee-off at a golf course that's often 50 kilometres away. I always hesitate though. We have slept apart for a few years now. He's a terribly light sleeper, and every twist and turn of mine in seeking some sort of comfortable balance disturbs him, so I always try to stay rigid as long as possible until an uncontrollable spastic jerk initiates a "Jesus" muttering; then I'll jolt out of bed and stumble down the hall to the spare bedroom where our daughter once slept, and there, I can thrash about as much as I like till I find peace.

My physiotherapist recently helped me find the perfect sleeping position: With my right side propped up against a crescent-shaped body pillow threaded between my knees, two soft pillows scrunched under my head and neck, and a small microbead cushion I stuff into the crevice of my lower back with my sentient fingers, the chronically angry areas on my left side from compensating for the strange "patterning" on my weakened side are given a relaxing reprieve. As well, with my right side buffered and still against the mattress, the stinging calms and recedes. In this position, I feel almost weightless.

This blissful sleeping pose often does not come without a lot of grunt work, but when the *Aha!* moment finally arrives, supreme drugged relaxation, deep breathing and sleep take over at almost the same moment my head sinks down.

And on a good night, I'll be in the same position when I open my eyes the next morning.

* * *

So, after tinkling at 4:30 a.m., still sleepy and comfortably numbed thanks to the nighttime dose of pregabalin and cannabis oil, I pad into the master bedroom, strip down and slip into bed next to Jean-Pierre. He is toasty hot, soft and welcoming, his kisses like sweet peaches, our arms and legs twining around each other, so content we are to be comfortably resting together. He quickly falls back into deep sleep by the time I gently turn away from him, and after he gets up, sometimes as early as 5:30 a.m., to make his hallowed first tee-off, wherever that may be, I can even return to nirvana, sometimes till around 7 a.m. …

Very rarely, but once in a while.

This particular morning, I dream that I am seated on a bench in a garden outside a medical clinic. It must be the Rehabilitation Centre. Many times, in real life, I would park far away and walk the beautifully treed paths leading to the complex, circled by a wooded area with a paved path, cement picnic tables and bird feeders.

But this time, I am crawling through the trees, and into a clearing. I discover a stack of shiny white, one-litre plastic containers; most of them are pristine, but a few are caked with bits of dried-up food waste and randomly scattered about. A matted, brown-knit shawl droops from a waist-high branch. I don't touch the dirty containers, but I gather up the clean stack and place it in a recycle bin next to the wide, sliding glass-doors at the entrance. I decide I better go back through the bushes to retrieve the wrap and bring it to the lost and found.

I arrive at the front desk, see the empty waiting room, and –

Oh my … with all your dithering in the bushes, you've probably missed your referral appointment, or whatever else you're here for … was it for the foot clinic, the brace, the Botox injections, the Chronic Pain Clinic assessment … ?

I try hard, but can't remember …

The glowing receptionist, completely clad in white, smiles sweetly and assures me there's no problem. *Dr. Mugabug is running late …* She takes the shawl I forget I'm holding. *It belongs to a homeless woman. She likes to sleep in the garden sometimes, but not to worry, she will come back for it …*

Another white coat stands off to the side of the counter. He looks tired but alert, with a mottled, grey crew cut, intently focussed on whatever he's reading. I recognize him, but can't remember his name.

Hey … weren't you the anesthesiologist for one of my surgeries?

He looks up quickly and smiles broadly.

Yes, I was … and I've been overseeing all of your procedures. How are you doing these days?

Quite well, thanks, all things considered …

He nods serenely. *Good, good … however, I have noticed your increasing addiction to object-matching and word games on your iPhone, in excess of six hours a day …*

I nod sheepishly. *Yes, I know … but with the pandemic and everything … it's SO much fun … and it distracts me from the pain … just like laughing … what should I do?"*

He closes his eyes and clasps his hands. *You already know what to do … get off your butt … go do Today's Walk… and keep on laughing …*

Yes, I know … independence … and almost never saying never … that's living …

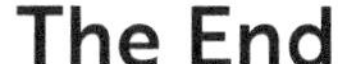

The End

Acknowledgements

I would never have made it to the finish line without the encouragement of so many writing doulas, starting with Traci Skuce, from Vancouver Island, B.C. Her benevolent guidance made me believe I could do things my own way. Traci's free online writer's summit in 2021 pointed me to a short but valuable conversation with New Zealand book coach Kathy Derrick, who fielded my questions and referred me to former New York Times journalist and writing coach Marion Roach. Marion's regular emails and author interviews helped me refine my craft. And finally, book doula Dallas Woodburn from San Francisco continues to cheer me on.

My husband and daughter helped me cut and strengthen so much copy, while my cherished pre-readers, Pascale Milne and Lucie Hemstead, helped me gain clarity.

Finally, The Self-Publishing Agency (TSPA) blessedly took the business reins from me to perform their marketing and production magic. In addition to the team headed by creative genius and CEO Megan Williams, COO Ira Vergani always kindly ensured no stone was left unturned in the production process, and Kathie Lynas, a seasoned journalist, teacher, writer and editor, was instrumental in helping make my story sing. The TSPA team provided me a safe haven, which allowed me to focus on my craft, without fear of rejection or wasting precious time. It's been just plain fun!

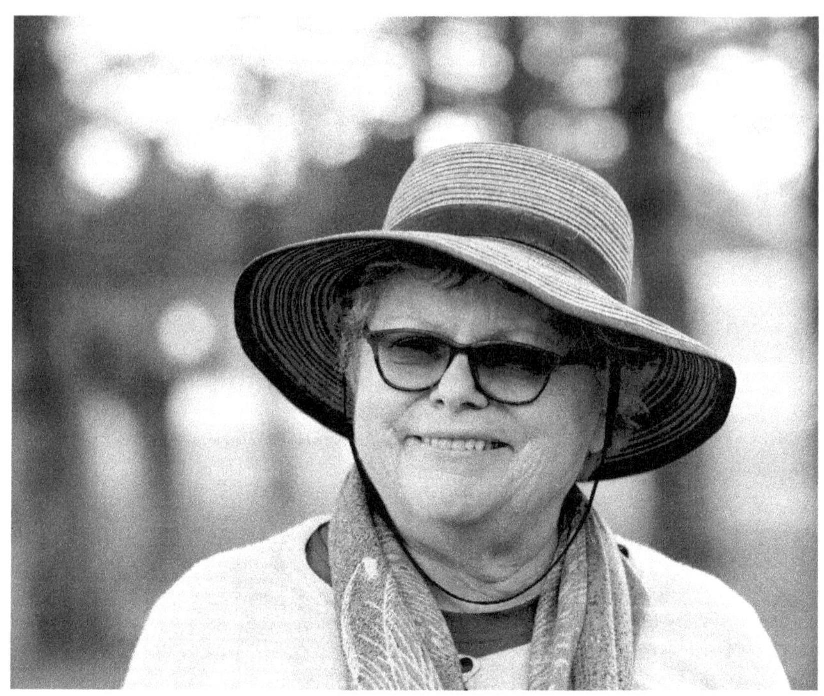

Photo: Geneviève Maurice Photography

About the Author

Cathy Allard was born in New Westminster, British Columbia and grew up in Canada's capital, Ottawa, Ontario. With a passion for writing and marketing, Cathy embarked on a career as a communications professional in the federal public service. Shortly after giving birth to her daughter, she found herself facing an unprecedented challenge – how to heal and eventually, thrive, after experiencing a stroke at the young age of 27.

Through rehabilitation and a setback after a second, more damaging stroke, Cathy was able to learn new ways to manage day-to-day living, motherhood and a return to her communications career, with experience working for such entities as Export Development Canada, the Secretary of State and Justice Canada. She was honoured to volunteer for several years with the Deputy Minister of Justice's Advisory Committee for Persons with Disabilities, where she shared her experiences and helped others with accommodation issues related to visible and invisible disabilities.

Now retired and a proud grandmother, Cathy currently lives in the Ottawa area with her husband, Jean-Pierre. She enjoys music, good food and gentle aquafit, and takes particular delight in walking, kayaking and snowshoeing.